"I have learned from experience that Crissa Constantine demonstrates the courage and the ability to abandon her wounds and learn to love herself. When you learn to love yourself and your life amazing things happen to your body."

Bernie Siegel, MD,
author of *Faith, Hope and Healing* and *A Book of Miracles*

"Brilliant and very emotional."

Laura Hesse, screenwriter and author of
The Holiday Series and *The Gumboot & Gumshoe Series*

"As more and more research shows connections between mental and physical health, Crissa demonstrates to the reader a framework of reexamining impressionable experiences of life. She shares her own challenges by taking the reader through vignettes and weaves her learnings of how she came to find her inner power of self-love. This book is a tool, for not only cancer patients but everyone, to discover the gift of self-love and acceptance."

Zoe Campbell,
professional fundraiser

"Crissa Constantine's book is a powerful message of hope and healing. Everyone who is struggling with a debilitating illness or an unhappy life will greatly benefit from reading her story of transformation. She beautifully and convincingly describes what true healing is all about and how you, too, can transform your life."

Gudrun Eichhorst,
Emotional Health Coach, The Oaktree Energy Medicine Center

"Illness, while never a welcome 'addition' to our world, often provides the impetus to search ourselves and, indeed, to search life itself more deeply and more passionately. In this beautifully written memoir, Crissa Constantine shares a remarkable journey of introspection, a journey that was in many ways launched as a result of an encounter with ovarian cancer. That this journey taught her that 'love has the last word' is reason indeed to celebrate, and to savour this account of her life and times."

Reverend Foster Freed,
Knox United Church, Parksville

"Crissa's stories remind us that life is full of transformative moments when we are willing to learn from the teachers we encounter along the way. Since reading her book, I have been more aware of what I say to others and to myself. This book issues the ultimate challenge—that we learn to be kind to ourselves."

Lisa Leger,
Women's Health Educator

"Beautifully written, with all sorts of interesting life stories, insights, and inspiration."

Brad Nelson,
Ph.D., Director,
Trev and Joyce Deeley Cancer Research Center, Victoria

Love and Accept Yourself Now

Love and Accept Yourself Now

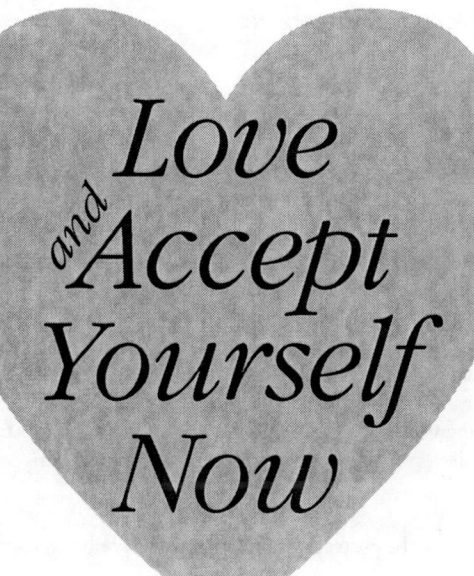

A Memoir

CRISSA CONSTANTINE

iUniverse, Inc.
Bloomington

Love and Accept Yourself Now
A Memoir

Copyright © 2012 by Crissa Constantine

All rights reserved. No part of this book may be used or reproduced by any means, graphic, electronic, or mechanical, including photocopying, recording, taping or by any information storage retrieval system without the written permission of the publisher except in the case of brief quotations embodied in critical articles and reviews.

Medical Disclaimer
The information, ideas, and suggestions in this book are not intended as a substitute for professional medical advice. Before following any suggestions contained in this book, you should consult your personal physician. Neither the author nor the publisher shall be liable or responsible for any loss or damage allegedly arising as a consequence of your use or application of any information or suggestions in this book.

iUniverse books may be ordered through booksellers or by contacting:

iUniverse
1663 Liberty Drive
Bloomington, IN 47403
www.iuniverse.com
1-800-Authors (1-800-288-4677)

Because of the dynamic nature of the Internet, any web addresses or links contained in this book may have changed since publication and may no longer be valid. The views expressed in this work are solely those of the author and do not necessarily reflect the views of the publisher, and the publisher hereby disclaims any responsibility for them.

Any people depicted in stock imagery provided by Thinkstock are models, and such images are being used for illustrative purposes only.

Certain stock imagery © Thinkstock.

ISBN: 978-1-4759-4768-7 (sc)
ISBN: 978-1-4759-4769-4 (hc)
ISBN: 978-1-4759-4770-0 (e)

Library of Congress Control Number: 2012915993

Printed in the United States of America

iUniverse rev. date: 09/24/2012

To all the angels in this world, and to all
those who yearn to love themselves

Contents

Preface xi
Acknowledgments xiii
Introduction 1

Part I

Chapter 1:   Cancer? Oh My God 7
Chapter 2:   Not Your Fault 16
Chapter 3:   Angels during Chemo 21
Chapter 4:   I Love You? 27

Part II

Chapter 5:   Ode to Joy 39
Chapter 6:   Mother Earth 47
Chapter 7:   Leroy 50
Chapter 8:   Desiree 59
Chapter 9:   The Rocket Scientist 78
Chapter 10: Venus 81
Chapter 11: Charles 86
Chapter 12: The Music of the Spheres 93
Chapter 13: Pierre and the Older Woman 97
Chapter 14: Ralph 109

Chapter 15:	Frank	113
Chapter 16:	Charmaine	119
Chapter 17:	Karma	158

Part III

Chapter 18:	Full of Hope	175
Chapter 19:	Third Chemo	183
Chapter 20:	Radiation	187
Chapter 21:	Through the Fire	196
Chapter 22:	An Attitude of Gratitude	199
Chapter 23:	Edward and Bianca	207
Chapter 24:	Corazon	214
Chapter 25:	Valentine's Day Every Day	224
Chapter 26:	Love Has the Last Word	234

Preface

I was diagnosed with invasive ovarian cancer in July of 2005 and had two major operations, three rounds of chemotherapy, and six weeks of radiation. The counseling I received during my chemotherapy treatments helped me to shed all of my negative, self-critical thoughts and paved the way toward total self-love and self-acceptance.

In 2008 I decided to share this wonderful feeling with others, so I wrote *Through the Fire*, a booklet about my experience with this silent killer, ovarian cancer. It was distributed to raise awareness and funds for early detection research and was greatly appreciated by cancer patients, cancer survivors, medical scientists, and some members of the general public. Nelly Auersperg, MD, PhD, an internationally praised ovarian cancer researcher who recently retired, said the booklet was excellent and should be distributed widely. Dr. Brad Nelson, an award-winning cancer researcher in Victoria, was very moved by it. Reverend Foster Freed of Knox United Church thought it was superb and said it was a healing template that could help others. Several members of the BC Cancer Foundation and the Canadian Cancer Society were happy I wrote the booklet, saying it could help a lot of people.

In 2011, I suddenly had the urge to transform the booklet into a full-length book and reach a wider audience because I know many people around the world need as much help as I did to learn to love and accept themselves 100 percent.

I had to face the deadliest of all the female cancers while living alone and without family support. A friend told me, "There must be a reason why you had to be so strong in your life." I didn't see the reason at first, but it has become clear to me. I have realized that if I would have had a family to help me through my cancer ordeal, I might have been too self-sufficient to reach out to the world and help others. Because of my experience, I see the whole world as my family and have a passionate need to help people disarm their inner critics so they can stand in front of a mirror and say, "I love you." When we can all do that, the world will be a much better place.

Acknowledgments

I would like to thank all of the medical researchers, doctors, and other health professionals who worked so hard to save my life. I was not ready to give up at fifty-four, and these last few years of my life have been the best yet!

I am very lucky to have met highly empathic counselors who helped me reach my goal of total self-love and self-acceptance.

Many of my good friends and acquaintances have been very supportive during my cancer journey, and I'm certain that their loyalty and constant prayers helped me recover.

Sheryl Cohn's book *The Boy in the Suitcase*[1] confirmed what I had always suspected. As a second-generation child of a refugee from Stalin's holocaust, I sometimes neglected my own emotional needs and tried too hard to protect my mother. My own battles and challenges in life seemed almost insignificant compared to hers, and that made it harder for me to concentrate on my own healing. The first step in solving a problem is to understand it, and I understand myself even more now.

Char Anderson is a terrific computer whiz who helped me organize the manuscript and send it to the editors at iUniverse.

I am very grateful to Krista Hill and the editors at iUniverse. Their suggestions for improving the manuscript were invaluable.

---

[1] Sheryl Cohn, *The Boy in the Suitcase: Holocaust Families Stories of Survival* (Lanham, MD: Hamilton Books, 2012).

Introduction

This book starts with a graphic description of my cancer diagnosis and a frank admission of the concomitant feelings of terror I experienced. I had to deal with a whole team of doctors and other health professionals, and I felt that my life was out of control.

In the chapter entitled "I Love You?" I discuss how my amazing counselor used Buddhism, empathy, intuition, and common sense to help me drop my negative emotional and mental baggage and begin the process of healing through self-love and self-acceptance. The mind-body connection is very strong, and one's chances of healing are much greater if one sends loving thoughts to every part of one's body. Most people have some harmful, self-critical thoughts that make their lives harder and more precarious than they have to be.

After my first round of chemotherapy, I analyzed my past to find the origin of my harsh inner critic. In "Ode to Joy," I reminisce about childhood bullying, parental neglect, and my longing for a kinder and less judgmental world. Through the process of analyzing my past, however, I also found the roots of my budding self-love and self-acceptance.

In "Mother Earth," I reminisce about a courageous and inspiring relative who was not accepted because she was poor. Nevertheless, she knew her own worth and demanded to be accepted for what she was.

I learned a lot from "Leroy," a poor black man who had enough compassion to save the world.

"Desiree" was a glamorous and enterprising friend who was not fully accepted by her family. She struggled very much with that rejection, and we would often console each other because we had similar problems.

"The Rocket Scientist" was a friend, but is also a symbol of so many incredibly brilliant people who don't fully love and accept themselves, no matter how accomplished they are.

"Venus" shows how competitive, jealous, and insecure some people can be when they don't accept themselves. I have met many people like that in my life, and this is just one example.

"Charles" was another accomplished, gifted man who felt he was not quite good enough, so he lashed out at others to make himself feel better. He wanted to marry me, but he was not always kind.

In "The Music of the Spheres," I write about a fantastic piano teacher who boosted my self-esteem.

"Pierre and the Older Woman" shows, among other things, how we glorify youth and dismiss the beautiful qualities of age. I cared very much for Pierre but felt that our relationship was doomed because I was a few years older than he was.

In "Ralph," I describe a troubled boy who found his life's purpose when he realized people loved and accepted him just as he was.

"Frank" was one of my brightest students, but he wasn't satisfied with that and joined a gang to prove that he was a tough macho man.

"Charmaine" was a godsend. She was a spiritually evolved nurse who helped me and my soul-damaged parents during a very critical time. She also became a unique friend who helped me through my cancer journey and strongly encouraged me to love and accept myself.

In "Karma," we see that unresolved childhood abuse can lead to cruelty and thoughts of suicide. Many of us need some professional help so we can learn to accept ourselves and others.

In "Full of Hope," I summarize some of what I learned from analyzing my past and discuss my spiritual growth as I underwent my second chemotherapy treatment.

"Third Chemo" shows how I reached my goal of total self-love and self-acceptance with the help of good counseling and loyal friends.

I actually looked forward to my radiation treatments because I wanted to heal completely and get rid of any residual cancer cells that might have been circulating in my body. I felt totally free after the treatments were finished and traveled extensively to celebrate being alive and to enjoy the present with greater passion and gusto than ever before.

When I went to a Bible study class after my cancer treatment was over, I learned that the image of Daniel being delivered through the fire is a symbol of what can happen in our present-day lives. This inspired me to write *Through the Fire,* my ovarian cancer awareness and fundraiser booklet.

Keeping a gratitude journal has greatly enhanced the quality of my life. By focusing on the positive aspects of every day and writing them down, one can improve one's attitude toward life. I have included a few journal entries as inspirational examples in "An Attitude of Gratitude."

The importance of love is the theme for the last three stories and the essay "Love Has the Last Word." I have written about Edward and Bianca, who had reasons to doubt their own self-worth, but they were lucky to meet, fall in love, and form a powerful, mutually healing relationship. And I was lucky to have met them when I was a little girl; they had a very positive influence on me in my formative years.

Ted was very bitter about his troubled past and couldn't enjoy life until he was overwhelmed by Corazon's love. I have met many people who are very much like Corazon and Ted.

"Valentine's Day Every Day" is the story of some wonderful, bighearted Americans and Canadians who live in El Salvador and who are helping the country and its orphans recover from a brutal civil war. They made an indelible impression on me.

In the essay "Love Has the Last Word," I attempt to show how pure logic, social research, medical research, and all the major religions point to the same conclusion: you have a right and a duty to love and accept yourself.

I was inspired to make sweet lemonade out of my cancer lemons, but you, dear reader, shouldn't have to face a deadly disease to wake up. I invite you to have a sip of my lemonade with the hope that it will improve your life.

Most of the names and initials and some circumstances in my stories have been changed to protect the innocent.

Part I

Chapter 1

Cancer? Oh My God

What is that blood doing on my pants? I'm almost fifty-four, and it's been well over a year since I had my last period. Is it a bit of harmless postmenopausal bleeding? Is it a benign fibroid? Mother had benign fibroids when she went through menopause, and she warned me to be prepared for trouble at this transitional time in my life. I wish I could discuss this with her, but she passed away just before Christmas. Now it's Easter, and I'm all alone.

I found the blood right after I came home from an Easter Sunday morning service at a nearby church. I didn't know what to think, so I ignored it and hoped it wouldn't return. When it reappeared a week later in early April 2005, however, I could no longer live in a state of denial and made an appointment to see my family physician.

His calm, thorough, and competent manner helped to soothe my frazzled nerves, but he ordered an abdominal ultrasound test just to be sure we weren't dealing with a serious condition.

I went to a nearby clinic, gave my doctor's requisition form to the receptionist, sat down, and waited for the ultrasound technician.

I had watched my mother have ultrasounds for gall bladder and liver problems, but I had never had the procedure myself. I wondered what it would feel like.

A pleasant-looking technician appeared after a few minutes and ushered me into a small room that had a computer and a chair placed next to a stretcher. She was very polite and soft spoken, and that made it easier for me to lie down and expose my abdomen so she could cover it with a warm gel. After I told her about my post-menopausal blood, she drew a sharp breath and said, "That's not always a good thing."

Oh no. I don't like the sound of that at all.

Even though the technician smiled as she moved a sensor device all over my abdomen to get a complete picture on the computer screen, I couldn't stop thinking about her words. *Not always a good thing, not always a good thing.* I wondered if my mom was looking down at me from the ceiling. She had been screened in that very room several years before. When the technician finished, she told me that the results would be read by a radiologist and then sent to my family physician.

My doctor called me a few days later and told me that the results showed what appeared to be a benign, fluid-filled ovarian cyst that is common with the typical monthly hormonal changes women have. These cysts can wax and wane every month and are usually perfectly harmless. I was very relieved to hear that, but I was also a bit confused. *But I am in menopause and have no more periods. What's going on?* I was told to go back to the lab for another ultrasound six weeks later because that was the standard procedure used to rule out the regular hormonal changes that can cause cysts.

In the meantime, I went on lots of long, rigorous hikes with my friends to try to distract myself from thinking too much about the cyst. It didn't work. No matter how beautiful the mid-Vancouver Island forests, rivers, waterfalls, and wildlife were, I was obsessed with the cyst. *Maybe it's cancer. But how can it be cancer? I can hike for two hours on forest trails without getting winded. It has to be a benign cyst. But is it really?*

I had my second ultrasound in May, and when I saw my doctor a few days later to hear about the results of the test, he looked quite concerned. "This time the cyst looks solid. It hasn't grown, but it doesn't just look fluid-filled anymore. It also has some thick nodules that weren't there before."

That sounds sinister. I don't like this at all. Maybe it really is cancer. What's going to happen to me?

He filled out some forms and several test orders. One of them was for a CA 125 blood test, which is used to detect proteins that may indicate the presence of ovarian cancer. I withered inside as I watched him write, "Cancer?" on one of the forms. "I'm going to refer you to Dr. A. He's a gynecologist and surgeon." I wasn't thrilled about that referral. I had never been examined by a gynecologist because I was single and had never had kids.

I was so nervous and anxious as I walked toward the gynecologist's office close to the hospital that my left leg seized up. *Why do I have to come here?* I opened the door, hobbled over to a chair, and sat down. I had to force myself to breathe. I had extra reasons to be nervous because I knew all the results from the tumor-marker blood tests my original doctor had ordered would be on Dr. A's desk; I must have looked as if I were about to be executed.

I didn't have to wait long before Dr. A appeared to usher me into his consultation room. He didn't smile, but he exuded great confidence as he asked me several questions about my lifestyle. We soon moved into the examination room, where he performed a complete pelvic exam. When he finished, he told me he couldn't feel any cyst. I was stunned. *Now what?* We moved back to the consultation room, and when I asked him about the numerous blood tests, he told me they were all negative.

I was immensely relieved to hear that, but I was still curious about the tests. "Which one is the most accurate?"

"The CA 125," he said with absolute certainty. It, like all the other tests, was negative. (A few weeks later, I learned that 15 percent of all women have blood that doesn't show evidence of immune activity against cancer cells. The blood tests are useless for those women. I happened to be one of those 15 percent.)

As relieved as I was to hear that the CA 125 test was negative, I was haunted by the second ultrasound that showed a thicker cyst with nodules and my family doctor's suspicion of cancer.

"I'm going to send you for another ultrasound, including a transvaginal ultrasound, just to make sure. It is possible that whatever is there may go away on its own. I'll only perform a laparoscopy to remove both ovaries if this third test shows a cyst. You might have a cystadenoma." He drew a little diagram to illustrate the laparoscopy procedure for me.

I looked at it and asked, "If the ovaries are removed, how will that affect my hormonal balance?"

"Not much. You may have a weaker libido; that's all." He shrugged.

The technician who performed the third test was quite friendly. She showed me the computer screen (even though technicians are not supposed to do that) and told me not to worry because the cyst on my left ovary, which looked like a blue-black hole, didn't have spots all around it. She explained that the dangerous cysts usually had spots around them, indicating an activated immune system trying to destroy cancerous cells. She also did the transvaginal ultrasound with a long, thin, lubricated apparatus.

A few days after the test, Dr. A told me I needed surgery and put me on the emergency list. I had turned fifty-four in May and had not had major surgery since I was two, when my tonsils were removed. *What next? My life is out of control.*

Even though I was shaking with fear on the stretcher in the operating room before the anesthetist worked his magic, the late-June morning surgery went well. I had to wear an uncomfortable urinary catheter, however, and those devices are notorious for allowing bacteria into the body.

A few days after I got home, I suffered extreme abdominal pain and was taken back to the hospital by ambulance. The pain was so intense that I needed lots of morphine. When I got home again, my legs became terribly swollen due to lymphedema and an anesthetic that might have caused a lazy colon. I looked like an elephant from the waist down. *Will the swelling ever disappear?*

In spite of the swelling, I was relieved because I had not heard from my family doctor for over two weeks. He told me he would call only if there was an emergency, and the results of the pathologists' analyses of the cyst were due back from the labs around July 10. It was already July 14, and it was 6:00 in the evening. *Would he call now, at suppertime? Of course he would. That is a preferred time for him to call patients, after his receptionists go home. Surely it's too late to call.*

Then the phone rang. *Oh, my God. It's him.* I knew it was him, even though I was sitting on my bed and my bedroom phone had no call display to identify who was calling. "Hello?" My voice was soft and weak.

"Hi, Crissa. The results just came back from the lab in Vancouver today." He sounded calm and caring, but I was terrified. "There was a slow-growing carcinoma in the cyst on your left ovary. I'm sorry to tell you over the phone, but I'm going on holiday tomorrow." I can't remember what I said, but he continued, "Dr. A will want to see you about this."

Dr. A was widely praised by other doctors as being a fantastic surgeon, and when he visited me after my operation, he told me the cyst looked basically benign when it was analyzed in the OR. I was so relieved to hear that as I was recovering from the operation. Both of my ovaries and Fallopian tubes were removed as a precaution, even though it was the left ovary that had the cyst. *And now this carcinoma bombshell from the pathologists?*

I couldn't speak right away. "If everything was removed, why do I have to see Dr. A?" I felt numb and my mouth was dry.

"Some of the cells got loose during the operation."

"Oh," I whispered as I began to tremble.

"Take care, and I'll see you later." He still sounded calm and caring, and that mollified my terror a little. I knew he was a very popular doctor, with an excellent reputation.

I called Dr. A's office the next day and made an appointment. Some good friends offered to accompany me, but I preferred to go alone. That might have been a mistake. My stomach was churning after the forty-minute drive, and I had to rush to a bathroom before I could face Dr. A.

I sat down in his office waiting area, hoping my stomach would give me peace.

Dr. A picked up my file at the receptionist's desk and led me into his office. He gave me a slight smile after we sat down across from each other. "You need a total abdominal hysterectomy."

My life is no longer my own, and I have no family to console me and give me courage. I have lots of friends but no family. It's horrible enough to have a cancer diagnosis, but to have to be at the mercy of strangers on top of that is almost diabolical. Dr. A continued to smile at me, and his fearless demeanor helped me face this nightmarish situation. I was truly grateful that he seemed to be the kind of doctor who can laugh at cancer. When one is so vulnerable, a fearless and defiant ally can make all the difference between life and death.

When I went to the hospital for a pre-op physical and blood tests a few days before the hysterectomy, a cheerful nurse examined me and gave me some brochures and pre-op information to read at home. I felt like weeping when I looked at the diagram of the female reproductive system. *What was the point of having all those organs? I never had the kids I wished I could have had, and now my whole system is going to be removed.* I wondered if I would still feel like a whole woman after the operation.

Two of my wonderful friends, a married couple, came to pick me up at 7:00 one beautiful August morning to take me to the hospital for my midmorning hysterectomy. I couldn't believe it, but I laughed when I saw them. Their two Bassett hounds, Molly and Stevie, emerged from the bushes dressed in hilarious outfits. Molly had shiny ruffles around her neck, making her look like a clown. Stevie, also a female, had a white cloth with a red cross on her back.

"That's Nurse Molly and Dr. Steve," they said.

The dogs trotted around the front yard and then hopped into the van that was parked in the driveway. I giggled all the way to the hospital as I watched the antics of the dogs beside me. They wouldn't sit still. They were climbing all over the seats like mischievous kids; no tranquilizers would have been as effective as those two dogs.

It was a good thing I had some comic relief on the way to the hospital, because as soon as I arrived in the surgical wing waiting area, a nurse gave me a form and a pen. I gasped sharply. The form indicated that the reason for my operation was *invasive cancer*. Then I knew—*this is no early-stage cancer.* It had already spread from the left ovary to my nearby reproductive organs, and that's why I needed a total hysterectomy and a removal of the omentum. Ovarian cancer cells apparently thrive in the omentum, a fatty layer close to the stomach. In spite of the fact that I had taken care of myself, had annual physicals for years, ate healthy foods most of the time, never smoked, had the occasional glass of wine, exercised regularly, and was not promiscuous, I had invasive cancer.

Another nurse appeared and beckoned me to the private area,

so I hugged my friend, thanked her for everything, and told her to thank her husband, who had stayed in the van with the dogs.

I was put on a stretcher in a waiting room, and an IV was started. The staff members were all very kind and sympathetic. I remembered the short trip to Hawaii I had taken in between operations. An adventurous friend had suggested I go to a place I'd never been before rather than just staying around town and worrying myself silly while waiting for the hysterectomy. I visualized the beach and the palm trees, trying to calm myself.

"I hope your family will be really supportive and help you during your recovery," a nurse said with genuine concern as I was wheeled into the OR.

"I don't have family here," I said.

"Oh, wow, that's awful." She looked at me with huge eyes.

"I know." I gave her a wan smile and thought about my mother's words of warning and that fateful Easter Sunday when I found the blood. It was as if she were urging me to take care of myself. In the meantime, I had found out that postmenopausal vaginal bleeding is often a symptom of ovarian cancer, and it's usually a sign of difficult-to-treat, advanced cancer. I was so grateful that my family doctor had ordered abdominal ultrasounds and that Dr. A had put me on the emergency list *again.*

Dr. A, my surgeon, appeared by my side in the OR. He was very kind and tried to soothe me while two anesthetists worked on my left hand. "Shall I call anyone?" he asked.

"No. My friends all know, and they'll be waiting for me …" I was thinking of Hawaiian beaches just before I went under.

Dr. A and his surgical assistant, a young lady doctor who was on her way to becoming a gynecologist, came to my room the next day after the operation. They had found abnormal masses deep within my pelvis and another abnormal mass attached to my rectum; they left that mass alone so they would not damage the rectum.

I was thunderstruck, but when Dr. A said, "Your chances of survival are high," I calmed down a little.

Then he said, "You're going to need chemo."

Oh my God.

"I'm going to be in charge of this," he said.

I was happy to hear that, because he was a fighter. He dismissed the cancerous cells as junk that had to be flushed out of an otherwise healthy body. He was like an angel who gave me the courage to face the next trial.

Chapter 2

Not Your Fault

In mid-September, a few weeks after my hysterectomy, I took an early-morning ferry and went to the BC Cancer Agency building next to the imposing Vancouver General Hospital to meet Dr. O, my gynecological oncology specialist. He is well known and writes protocols for cancer treatments. I didn't have to wait very long before a receptionist called me into the private office area. I liked Dr. O right away because he was very polite and warm, had a sense of humor, and inspired confidence. We had a short conversation, and then he left the examination room so I could undress and put on a hospital gown. I changed quickly and then sat on the examination table. *I was born in this hospital, and here I am, half naked and completely vulnerable, wondering if my days are numbered or if I'll have a second chance to start a new life.*

After a few minutes, he returned with a young intern at his side and then examined me gently and very thoroughly. I was apprehensive, but he didn't find any evidence of tumor recurrence and discussed the manual exam with the serious and soft-spoken intern.

"You may be cured right now because of the two operations, but you may have microscopic cancer, which can be fatal. That's why we strongly suggest that you go ahead with the chemo and the radiation. Dr. A is an excellent surgeon, but even he wouldn't be able to save you from microscopic cancer. The three rounds of chemo can be done in Nanaimo, and then we'll see you back here for the radiation portion of the treatment. Do you have any questions?" he asked, speaking with professorial authority.

"Yes! I've been reading lots of books about cancer, and many people think there's a cancer personality. They think that those who get cancer are 'type-C' personalities—people who are unassertive and look after others more than themselves. I was a caregiver for both parents because I'm an only child, but no one has ever called me weak. Almost everyone who knows me says I'm really strong. Trudeau was strong and got cancer, and Hans Selye was strong and got cancer," I said emphatically.

He was just as emphatic. "Personality has nothing to do with it. Strong people get cancer just as often as weaker ones." I was relieved to hear that because I didn't want to think of myself as weak or unassertive.

"I'm glad to hear that! I've been trying to psychoanalyze myself lately, but I always come up with the same conclusion: I may have had my setbacks, but I'm ambitious and assertive and that's why I earned lots of degrees. I looked after my parents for years because they were helpless and I felt sorry for them. In fact, people who knew us wondered where I found the strength to do that. Many of them said they wouldn't have been able to endure caregiving for any length of time. What about having a positive attitude about recovery? Even neighbors tell me they've heard that's supposed to make a big difference." I looked at him hopefully.

He shook his head. "I don't think it does. I've seen miserable people get better." We both had a good laugh. "It's true," he said.

"Did I get this because I didn't have kids? I've heard that can be a reason."

"Not necessarily. We think that the cells on the surface of the ovary can get confused because they have to divide more than other tissues in the body, and sometimes they just don't know when to stop. You did nothing wrong. It's not your fault. I read the report from Nanaimo, and apparently you've never smoked and only have the occasional glass of wine."

"That's true. I've never taken drugs either. I've been exercising for years, I use olive oil for cooking, I avoid red meat and ice cream and things like that, and I take multivitamins. Oh! What about my electric keyboard? I play that a lot because my grand piano is very loud, I don't want to disturb the neighbors at night, and I like privacy when I compose. Is the field around it dangerous?"

"I haven't heard anything about that, and ovarian cancer was around long before keyboards were invented," he replied.

"I guess I'm going to lose my hair during chemo," I said while touching my shoulder-length hair.

"Oh, yes, you will. Whenever I see a woman with your length of hair, I always think, *She's going to miss that.* Men will also shun you because they think your disease is contagious."

I just chuckled. *That doesn't matter. Mr. Right hasn't shown up yet anyway.*

Then I remembered the times when I was recovering from both operations in the hospital; after each operation, I was given a questionnaire that asked if I had suffered a recent loss. My mother had passed away just a few months before I was diagnosed, and even though she was deeply troubled and had asked her doctor for an abortion when she was pregnant with me, I was deeply attached to her. We were very close. My financial advisor also told me that he had noticed that surviving spouses often get cancer just months after the death of their partners. In fact, several people have noticed the same thing, but it's difficult to prove a causal relationship. I didn't feel like asking him about this.

"I'll leave now, and Dr. R, the radiation oncologist, will be here soon. Sorry about having to start the radiation during the holiday season, but we don't want to wait more than a month after your last chemo in November."

Dr. O walked out with the intern, and I just stayed on the examination table. I thought about the endless sleepless nights I had suffered through during perimenopause and menopause and wondered if my hormonal imbalance that didn't allow me to sleep had weakened my immune system so much it became ineffective against cancer cells. Zopiclone, a prescription sleeping pill many women use during menopause, was useless for me. I was frequently up most of the night and then had to crash in the afternoon and have a nap. Sometimes I had so much energy I didn't even need a nap after only one hour of sleep at night. It was incredible.

No one is supposed to survive that kind of sleep deprivation for very long, but I carried on like that for months and months. Acupressure and massage didn't help much, and homeopathic medicines were useless. Sometimes I swam and hiked for hours, hoping I'd be tired enough to sleep, but it didn't work. A little bit of natural progesterone rubbed on my skin (recommended by some doctors) was the only thing that sometimes worked. I *never* took conventional hormone replacement therapy (HRT) because I knew about the frequent, serious side effects.

The radiation oncologist came in and introduced himself. His pleasant manner made me feel at ease as he shook my hand. "I'll be honest: radiation can cause a secondary cancer, but the chances of the ovarian cancer coming back are much bigger than that. You'd be wise to go ahead with the six weeks of radiation." He sounded very convincing.

"When do I start that?"

He looked on the wall calendar. "In mid-December, about a month after your last round of chemo." He already knew about the September, October, and November chemo sessions that had been set up for me at the Nanaimo hospital cancer clinic.

"If it might save my life, what can I do?" I said, shrugging.

He gave me a knowing smile and waved as he left.

I got dressed and went to another office in the cancer agency to pick up some brochures and booklets about ovarian cancer, chemo, and radiation, and the clerks told me I would be getting a research questionnaire in the mail. Some doctors were trying to see if there was a connection between lifestyle and ovarian cancer.

After I got home, I placed the brochures and booklets in my kitchen close to the phone. I didn't feel like reading them right away because I was already overwhelmed by my precarious situation and couldn't concentrate enough to absorb any more information. The questionnaire arrived a couple of days later; it was very long and detailed, with questions about all the jobs I ever had, my eating habits, my personal hygiene habits, and several other things. I filled it out and mailed it back right away.

A few days later, I met a lady who had suffered through ovarian cancer when she was only in her early thirties. She said her friends and family told her, "Oh, you got that because you're promiscuous."

I gave a little sarcastic laugh. "Yeah, right. You can live like a nun and still get it. It's not your fault."

"I know," she said. We hugged each other tight. We knew we didn't deserve to be judged.

Chapter 3

Angels during Chemo

I saw Dr. A in September, several days before my first round of chemo and he told me that some of the pathologists had classified my cyst as Stage IIIa. He had absolute confidence that it was curable, and that was very reassuring. Several pathology reports also came back completely negative for any malignant cells that might have been circulating in my abdomen. That was even more reassuring. However, I was shocked when he told me that the decision makers in the cancer agency would not have recommended chemo treatments if I had been in my seventies and had a heart condition. I was "only fifty-four," so they decided to go ahead with the chemo. *I guess some people are too old for all that expensive chemo? Each round costs thousands of dollars.* Again, I realized how little control I had over my own destiny. My life depended on the whims of strangers, and I felt as powerless as a foot soldier in an army full of generals. I resented it. I *hated* it.

I met the doctor in charge of chemo in the cancer clinic at the Nanaimo hospital a few days before my first round. He seemed pleasant enough and told me I had a 70 percent chance of surviving without chemo and that chemo only helps in a small percentage of cases. He was hoping I would be in that small percentage and that my chances of survival would be boosted up to 85 percent after the chemo. I thumbed through the thick pathology report package. One report had the words "evidence of uterine malignancy," and that confirmed the hysterectomy pre-op form that described my cancer as invasive.

The clinic's staff members were all very kind and supportive, and they set up a pre-chemo video session for me. I was pleased to get brochures detailing all the support services available to me, including nutritionists and counselors. I would be getting regular blood tests to check my platelet levels and to make sure my immune system wasn't too disabled during the treatments. I was warned to stay away from people with colds and was advised to eat lots of good protein. I was also told to avoid sharp objects because cutting yourself when your platelet count is low is very dangerous because you can bleed uncontrollably.

One morning in the third week of September, on the day of my first chemo session, I sat in a comfortable padded chair and looked at several other chemo patients who were already hooked up to the IV bags. A nice nurse with a soft voice explained to me that an anti-nausea drug would be injected for half an hour before the actual chemo treatment. The cancer clinic doctor had previously warned me that a few people are severely allergic to these drugs but that the staff would stop the treatment immediately if an allergic reaction began to occur. *Am I going to be allergic? If so, what will I feel like? Will I have seizures? Will I have trouble breathing?*

The nurse put a needle in a vein close to my wrist and started the drip. I looked up at the bag and wondered if it was poison. A volunteer came by and put a blanket in my lap. My muscles tightened up all over, and I wanted to jump out of the chair and walk around the room to relieve the tension. Fortunately, that was my only reaction to the drug, and it was mainly psychological.

"You don't seem to be allergic," the nurse said. "Good. We can continue. After half an hour, we'll start the chemo, and that will last for about four hours."

"We've got magazines and papers if you want them. I'll be right here," the friendly volunteer who had given me the blanket said. In spite of the fact that I was relieved not to have an allergic reaction, my muscles stayed very tense, and I had a terrible time sitting still. I kept shifting in my chair, wishing I could get up and walk. That lasted the whole four hours it took to complete the treatment!

"Take your time getting up," a motherly nurse said when the treatment finished. "Don't rush, in case you get dizzy."

"Amazingly enough, I'm not dizzy," I said.

"Do you have a ride home? Remember, you're not supposed to drive today at all."

"Yeah, I'll call my friend on her cell. She said she'd go shopping around here so she wouldn't be too far away when I called. Hey, I'm not even nauseated yet. I've heard so much about the nausea that most patients get, but I don't have it yet." I tried to sound brave.

"Good! Remember to ask your friend to help you fill your prescriptions on the way home. You'll need more antinausea medication. And remember to call if you have any problems at all. There's always a cancer specialist on call, even if it's in Victoria. And if you have to come to the emergency room here, show them your ID card so they can see you're on chemo."

I called my friend, and she came to pick me up within minutes. We stopped at a pharmacy, and then she took me home. "Call me if you need anything," she said.

"Thanks for everything," I said as I waved good-bye.

I went into the house and had a short nap. When I got up, I perused the notes I made while watching the video I was shown before the chemo and then looked at the brochures and booklets about ovarian cancer because I had more time to study them now and felt I could finally concentrate enough to learn something new.

Suddenly I felt as if I had been stabbed in the stomach with an ice pick. "No! No!" I screamed.

One of the booklets indicated that the prognosis for women diagnosed with Stage III cancer was very poor. *I was Stage III.* Here I was in my beautiful kitchen with a partial view of the ocean and the glaciers on the mainland, and I couldn't enjoy it. I felt as if I had just read my own death sentence. I screamed again and again and again.

This can't be happening. But what about the doctors who told me I had high chances of survival? Please, please, I hope they were right. You can't believe everything you read. You have to go with what the doctors told you. Forget about this. Forget about it. You can't live with that kind of fear. You don't deserve that.

I put the booklet back in the folder and sat by the phone. I wanted to call a crisis counselor. Then I remembered a friend who is a computer expert and also a writer and counselor. I called him and left a message.

He called me back after supper and agreed to come to my house and discuss a counseling plan. He was very sympathetic and completely understood my panic. I held my head in my hands for a long time after I closed the phone. *I'm too young to die. I'm not ready yet. I'll do anything it takes to survive this and have some quality years after this ordeal is over.*

I called a phone psychic in the evening and spoke about my extreme anxiety.

"You're going to be okay. Believe it or not, the worst is behind you," the psychic said.

We talked for about ten minutes, and I felt better. Then I realized how desperate this really was. I remembered all those university science courses I had taken and reminisced about the science program I designed at a school in California. Many of my students won awards for their science projects. I wondered what they would have said if they could have heard me asking for reassurance from a phone psychic. *Be easy on yourself. You're alone and desperate.*

Even though Dr. O, the gynecological oncologist in Vancouver, did not think there was a correlation between personality and cancer, I had a strong suspicion that my dysfunctional family life might have contributed to an immune system breakdown. I felt an overwhelming need for counseling, and I trusted my computer friend, C, because he had been severely abused as a very young child. His mother didn't want him, and he could already feel that while he was in her womb. Then his mother gave him away to his violent grandparents. Instead of becoming bitter and dangerous, however, he grew up to be an unusually compassionate man with tremendous insight into the human condition.

I also remembered a professor of psychology who told me that people who have been betrayed and abandoned in childhood and experience abandonment again in adulthood are very often diagnosed with either cancer or heart disease within seven years of the adult abandonment. That happens if the childhood trauma is unresolved. Some people never get the counseling they so desperately need, and others get it when it's almost too late. I wasn't sure if that was valid because I grew up in a medical family and didn't think that psychologists (who are not medical doctors) would know much about physical diseases like cancer and heart disease. However, this thought preyed on my mind. *Could this be true?*

I had also visited a counselor at a mental health center to try to cope with my mother's extreme alcoholism and was told that children who come from dysfunctional families often overextend themselves in an effort to fix their family problems. The counselor was not surprised that I had sacrificed a good deal of my life as a caregiver. Some health professionals have noticed a strong correlation between caregiving and a weakening of the immune system.

Before C's first visit, I went to my church for a session of healing touch. I had heard from friends how wonderful these sessions were and thought this was the time to try them. To receive healing touch, one lies down on a stretcher and two people, both of whom are trained in healing touch, stand on either side of you and ask you where the trouble spots in your body are. Then they appear to work on the energy field above the trouble spots and move their hands over your body without actually touching it.

I was very comforted while two lovely ladies worked on the area above my abdomen. They spoke soothing words and asked me to think of Jesus, who apparently practiced healing touch. A retired minister trained these ladies. Both of the ladies felt that I had a lot of internal healing energy in that area. No matter what one says about the theory of this practice, it was a beautiful experience, and that's what counts.

"I brought this for you. I knew you were coming," one of the ladies said as she presented me with a little gold angel pin. "You've been called upon to be amazingly strong in your life's journey. I hope this angel will protect you always." She spoke as if she were the best friend I ever had.

I thanked her and pinned it on my sweater as she gave me a sweet smile.

Chapter 4

I Love You?

C came to my house one morning a few days after my first round of chemo, and I told him about the last twelve years of my life. My father had suffered a massive stroke in the right hemisphere of his brain, rendering him more or less paralyzed on the left side of his body. He could at least think and talk, making it easier for my mother and me to cope with him. However, doctors were amazed that he lasted five and a half years after a stroke that almost always killed people immediately or turned them into vegetables. Dad was known for his iron will and incredible persistence in the face of disaster. I looked after him for three years and three months at home, but he had to be placed in a nursing home for the last couple of years of his life because he developed congestive heart failure on top of all of his other health problems.

My mother had her own serious health issues and dealt with Dad's stroke by drinking heavily and sometimes acting like a violent teenager. She often beat Dad while he was laying down, and I would have to pull her away from him. Once I even had to drag Dad to the victims' services section of the police station. A geriatric care nurse who was sent to our house by a concerned doctor thanked me for taking Dad to the police, saying that made it easier for her to place him on an emergency list for a nursing home.

I went to Al-Anon meetings to try to understand Mom's severe problem, and one of the things I found most useful was the Al-Anon book, *Courage to Change*.[2] According to this book, you're supposed to let your loved ones face the consequences of their drinking and still love them just the same. *You can't change another person; all you can do is change yourself and your own attitude.*

After several visits to our house, the geriatric care nurse said she thought I was ready to pull my hair out and looked as if I was fit to be tied. While we talked on the driveway, safely out of earshot of my mother, she told me she didn't know how I could stand living in such an incendiary atmosphere. She also said the psychiatrist she reported to was apparently infinitely more worried about me than he was about my parents.

I also told C about my life *before* I became a full-time caregiver.

"How long have you been suppressing your true nature?" C asked me with an intensely inquisitive look. He was comfortably seated on the living room couch across from me.

I thought about it for a while. "A long time," I admitted.

"How long? Exactly how long?" he persisted.

I hesitated. "I guess most of my life. Fifty-four years?" It seemed unbelievably long.

He nodded. "From the way you've described your life so far, that's right. That's one hell of a long time." Then he jumped up from the couch. "Let's go to the bathroom mirror." He motioned in that

---

[2] *Courage to Change: One Day at a Time in Al-Anon II* (New York, Al-Anon Family Group Headquarters, 1992).

direction, and we were soon standing in front of it. "I want you to look at yourself—I mean *really* look at yourself."

"Okay," I said as I sheepishly smiled at my own image.

"Now tell yourself how much you love yourself. Go on, say it." He spoke in an urgent tone, as if my life depended on it.

I stared at myself for several seconds. "I love you?" I said with a wavering voice. It felt very unnatural to say that, and I was embarrassed.

"I want you to say that to yourself every thirty minutes every day from now on, whether you're standing in front of the mirror or not. Learning to love and accept yourself is the main attitude change you need to make. You're already doing well. I knew some people who lost the will to live after they were diagnosed. They just gave up, and they died a few weeks later. You want to live, but you have to learn to accept yourself just the way you are. You're perfect just the way you are." His voice was strong and clear.

"I am?" I looked at him with wide eyes. "If you say so." I shrugged and gave a shy smile.

"You've got a lot of anger too, and it's a healthy type of anger that comes from self-defense. However, you don't have strong boundaries." He was blunt.

"I don't?" I frowned.

"Let's do an experiment. I'll show you what I mean." We walked out of the bathroom and into the hallway. "You stand right here, and then I'll walk ten paces behind you and stop. Then I'll start walking toward you, and I want you to raise your hand when you think I've come too close to you." He walked toward me and almost bumped into me because I couldn't feel his approach until the very last minute. "See what I mean? You've allowed your boundaries to be too porous."

We tried the experiment several times in several different ways, and I eventually understood the meaning of it all. I got better and better at sensing his proximity and seeing how the activity related to encounters with other people. If you really love yourself, you don't let others walk all over you. You develop a strong sense of personal space and don't allow it to be easily violated. This experiment was a powerful symbol of my real life.

After the experiment, we sat down and discussed happiness. It has nothing to do with the mind or intellect or a high IQ. It is a dynamic that originates in the heart, and to find true happiness, one has to move away from the head and into the heart. One has to connect with one's true nature and stop analyzing everything so much. We sometimes get so preoccupied with fearful thoughts that we can't enjoy life and get too far removed from our true spirits. C told me to think of my heart as the center of my existence and to repeat these phrases several times a day:

"I am whole. I am complete. I am perfect just as I am."

True healing can only come when we reconnect with the life force within us. He suggested I buy several books, including Jack Kornfield's *A Path with Heart*.[3] He also insisted that I start a journal, because that is supposed to be excellent for healing. I had heard the same thing from a breast cancer survivor.

C counseled me for almost two hours and told me he would return in a few days. I thanked him and started a journal as soon as he left. I enjoyed keeping a journal and found it to be very therapeutic. I also looked at myself in the mirror every thirty minutes and said, "I love you." It felt better and better to say that as the days passed but still rather strange and unnatural.

I bought Jack Kornfield's book and loved every page of it. Dr. Kornfield is an internationally renowned teacher, psychologist, and meditation master who grew up in a scientific and intellectual family and went to an Ivy League college. He said that he was

---

[3] Jack Kornfield, *A Path with Heart* (New York: Bantam Books, 1993).

surrounded by many bright and creative people who were unhappy in spite of their success and intellectual attainments. He realized that intelligence and worldly position had little to do with happiness or healthy human relationships. Because he was lonely and confused, he turned to Eastern wisdom and spirituality.

In the Buddhist tradition, all life is precious, and the important question at the end of one's life is: "Did I live my path with heart?" Love is the most important force in our lives, and one should bring loving-kindness to wounds and illness. That encouraged me to send loving thoughts to my body during my healing process and not to blame myself or feel guilty for being a cancer patient.

There are many beautiful guided meditations in the book, and the end of the first chapter has some very powerful words of wisdom: "You begin with yourself because without loving yourself it is almost impossible to love others."[4]

My counselor came back a few days later with a copy of Stephen Levine's *A Gradual Awakening*.[5] Levine stresses that everyone has a sense of unworthiness to some degree, and we carry it around with us like a cloud. It blinds us to our own beauty and is the result of being conditioned out of trusting our natural being. Too many of us have a critical, judging voice commenting on what we're doing and how we're doing it, pointing out that we're not coming up to par and are not worthy of love. We have somehow come to think that it's not appropriate to love ourselves—that we're not worthy of self-love—because we have lost our natural love of ourselves and our natural self-respect.

We are worthy of letting go of our unworthiness. The more we accept of ourselves, the more fully we experience the world. The more we accept our anger, our loneliness, and our desire systems, the more we can hear others and ourselves.

---

[4] Ibid., 20.
[5] Stephen Levine, *A Gradual Awakening* (New York: Anchor Books, 1989).

Another friend gave me a copy of Dr. Bernie Siegel's classic book *Love, Medicine, and Miracles*.[6] Dr. Siegel says he cannot overemphasize the importance of learning to love oneself and others. The truth is that love heals, and unconditional love is the most powerful known stimulant of the immune system. I was shocked when I read that 80 percent of his patients (he was a famous cancer surgeon before retiring to write inspirational books) were unwanted or treated indifferently as children. Kids who grow up knowing they're not wanted have a lifelong feeling of unworthiness and often develop cancer as a way out of a life without love. *The fundamental problem most patients face is an inability to love themselves because they have been unloved by others during some crucial part of their lives.*

I had read Christiane Northrup's book *The Wisdom of Menopause*[7] before my diagnosis. After I was diagnosed, I read it again with a deeper understanding of our unity of mind, body, and spirit and the connection between emotional health and physical health. Dr. Northrup emphasizes the importance of early life experiences and how they shape adult behavior. If you want to have more successful relationships in life, you must analyze your past to see what forces are driving you.

When I started my journal, I wrote about how I would criticize myself too often. Almost everyone is guilty of some harmful, excessive self-criticism. *Why are you so absentminded? Stop acting like a baby. Why can't you lose those extra ten pounds? Who died and left you in charge?* I was born with a strong personality and an intense need for freedom. I developed an intense desire to achieve early in life, but I often felt that I had not done enough in life. Even though I was happy that

---

[6] Bernie S. Siegel, *Love, Medicine, and Miracles* (New York: HarperCollins, 1998).
[7] Christiane Northrup, *The Wisdom of Menopause* (New York: Bantam Books, 2012).

I had integrity and lots of friends, I probably only loved myself about 80 percent. Most of us are conditioned to criticize ourselves from early childhood—probably so we won't become too selfish to contribute to society. The needs of the individual are subjugated for the sake of the group. That's an idea with good intentions, but when the subjugation of the self is carried too far, it becomes terribly harmful. Then some of us have to spend a lot of time and money trying to become whole again—trying to love and accept ourselves enough so we can be fully functioning members of society.

Whenever I stood in front of the mirror to say, "I love you," I realized that I didn't love myself 100 percent. It was painfully obvious. When I was a student, some men resented me for not being "easy" and told me I was too proud and too selfish. Some even told me I should have been "thrown in a haystack and gang raped to be shown what it is to be a woman." Some people told me I was lazy, others told me I was vain, and some told me I had no life or willpower of my own and was controlled by my parents. Some people told me they admired classical music but that I was wasting my time studying it because it was impossible to make money with it. These cruel judgments did not actually destroy me, but they lived in my brain like tiny demons with cynical little voices.

As I analyzed myself, I realized that my cancer had at least one silver lining: it was a great excuse to start trying to love myself profoundly and treating myself as a holy vessel. No one could predict exactly how much time I had left, but I wanted to aim for the highest possible quality of life! I began to feel what C was telling me—that the mind generates these feelings of inadequacy. He urged me to move away from my mind and into my heart.

You carry the cure within your own heart, and your heart knows you're lovely and loveable just the way you are. Whether you have cancer or not, you have an excuse to fully love and accept yourself. Life is too short to live any other way.

In *Boundaries*, Dr. Henry Cloud and Dr. John Townsend[8] say that our lives are a gift from God, and our spiritual and emotional growth is God's interest on his investment in us. When we say no to people and activities that are hurtful to us, we are protecting God's investment, so we have a right and a duty to avoid people who make us feel uncomfortable and appear to be toxic to us.

Not everyone will be sympathetic toward a cancer patient. One acquaintance told me that I got ovarian cancer because I didn't produce children, and this was nature's way of getting rid of me. Others told me my days were numbered and that my life would deteriorate after the cancer.

I enjoy watching Wayne Dyer on public television. He frequently talks about the beautiful source energy that makes our lives possible and says that positive people can help you connect with that energy. Negative people are to be avoided.

Soon after my first round of chemo, all my hair fell out. I would find gobs of it on my pillow, and one day a neighbor asked me into his house and shaved off the rest of the stubble. I wanted to make the best of this situation, so I went to a special hair salon and tried some wigs. The hairdresser and I picked a sophisticated gray-blonde Raquel Welch shoulder-length wig. It looked good, and I enjoyed wearing it because it reminded me of my younger days. I also bought some lovely shawls and used them as turbans. People often stopped me in the street to tell me how nice they looked.

I wore the wig and often stood in front of the mirror to say, "You're looking great, and you've got a great spirit. I love you more and more each day." I began to shed my harmful, negative baggage and my airtight ego and felt that I was just an infinitesimally tiny part of the biosphere and the universe.

---

8   Henry Cloud and John Townsend, *Boundaries* (Grand Rapids, MI: Zondervan, 1992).

As a musician, I love the idea that every living thing is a member of a cosmic symphony or choir. We should all work together to produce the heavenly masterpiece of life. Is the French horn superior to the violin? Is the clarinet superior to the bass drum? Is the soprano superior to the baritone? There should be no judgment at all. All cosmic instruments, including humans and all other living things, are unique and invaluable and should be treated as such.

There are so many images that can help us feel that we are integral parts of the human family and the cosmos, and here are a few:

- We are all leaves on the same tree.
- We are all petals on the same flower.
- We are cells in the same body.
- We are the tiny raindrops that refract sunlight and form rainbows.
- We're all just slightly different patterns of the same DNA.
- We're all snowflakes with different configurations.
- We're just another water molecule in the ocean.
- We're grains of sand on a long beach.
- Each one of us is a piece of the seven billion–member jigsaw puzzle that paints a picture of mankind.
- We're all connected through Jung's collective unconscious mind.
- We're different words in the same book.
- We're just specks of cosmic dust.

I was transformed by this feeling of connectedness, as if I were performing surgery on myself and removing a rusty nail from my brain or repairing a broken wing so I could fly again. I was like a butterfly emerging from a chrysalis or a traveler arriving at an airport and leaving useless old baggage on the tarmac before boarding a plane to heaven.

I kept analyzing my life to fully understand why it took some practice to tell myself, "I love you!" I also thought about why it was so difficult for so many *other* people to say that to themselves. Some of the people I met were brilliant while others were average. Some were gorgeous, and some were plain, but most of them did *not* fully love and accept themselves, and their lives reflected that sad truth.

However, a few I met loved themselves so totally that they radiated light wherever they went. I thought about how lucky I was to have met some of these spiritually evolved angels in my journey; my life would have been much harsher without them.

Part II

Chapter 5

Ode to Joy

I was sent to Athens to stay with my grandmother right after I finished first grade in Vancouver. A doctor had told my parents that I had to be sent to a warmer, dry climate for a while because I was in danger of contracting tuberculosis. My mother was exhausted because I was always sick, and my father was too busy with his medical research to help her look after me. Even though I already knew some Greek from my first visit there, a tutor helped me get ready to attend grades two and three in a Greek elementary school. Adults treated children with tenderness and affection at that time in Greece, and my teachers were extremely patient and soft spoken. My fellow students were generally quite gentle and kind as well; I don't remember any bullying or cruelty.

I missed my parents very much, however, and wondered why I was put on a plane by myself and sent so far away. I knew the ostensible reason, but on some deeper level, I felt guilty for having chronic bronchitis and being such a burden to them. I liked my grandmother, my stepgrandfather, and my half uncle, but I felt that I was being punished for being physically fragile.

Luckily, there were enough distractions everywhere around me to suppress my frustrations.

I had been taken up to the Parthenon when I was four, but I didn't care for it, saying, "There were too many stones." On this second prolonged visit, however, I was transfixed by the ubiquitous stone ruins in the city and in the countryside and would often daydream about living in ancient times. I loved the schoolbook drawings and stories about the twelve Olympian gods, the famous figures from the *Iliad* and the *Odyssey*, and all the other mythological characters. I had a special respect for the ones like Hephaestus (also known as Vulcan), who toiled night and day to make tools for the other gods.

Drawings of two mythological women in particular made a permanent impression on me. One lady looked outrageously flamboyant, with a mane of long, dark hair, lots of flashy jewelry, plenty of vivid makeup, scarlet red lips, and a long, spangled, flaming red dress. The other lady, who appeared next to her, looked very demure, with plain hair and no makeup or jewelry, and she wore a simple long white dress. Our teacher told us that the lady in red represented vulgar materialism, selfishness, shallowness, and an unquenchable desire for power over others. The lady in white, on the other hand, represented the kinder virtues of altruism, self-sacrifice, true love for your fellow man, compassion, and nobility of soul.

I immediately connected with the lady in white and wanted to be like her. I often imagined that our school was burning and that I was the pilot of a magical flying machine and that I would swoop down and save all my schoolmates and teachers from the horrific inferno. I had an overwhelming need to help mankind, as if we really were all brothers and sisters, and it gave me tremendous joy to daydream about it.

As much as I was mesmerized by the ruins all around me, they reminded me of the near obliteration of the Greek people after four hundred years of Turkish oppression. The grownups told me stories about daily life in Greece in those days. If the Greeks didn't prostrate themselves before a Turkish pasha, they risked being beheaded with a scimitar on the spot. Now, as an adult, I see this as one of the end results of our compulsion to cruelly bully and judge others. *You're not one of us, so we chop your head off.* The same intolerant types would send innocent victims to Auschwitz or Siberia or hijack planes and fly them into skyscrapers.

When my grade-three teacher told my classmates I was going back to Canada on the last day of class before the summer holidays, all the boys and girls lined up to hug and kiss me and to say goodbye. Those two lonely years in Greece helped to expand my mind and spirit, but they did not prepare me for the return to the fast-paced world of Vancouver.

"Come on, get out of bed! You have to go to school," my mother said anxiously.

"I don't want to, Mum. Everyone is so mean to me there," I whined. It was the second week of grade four back in Vancouver, and I was suffering from severe culture shock. Even though I was happy to be reunited with my parents, they were both impatient with me for not adjusting quickly to my new life. They didn't seem to understand how difficult it was for me to think like a modern Canadian again after living in a country that dwelled on its ancient history. I felt that I must have done something bad and deserved to be mistreated.

Mom dragged me out of bed, and I reluctantly got dressed. She gave me breakfast and drove me to school. I hated to see her drive off and leave me behind in a pool of sharks. Even though English was my first language, I had been speaking Greek for two years and was hesitant about speaking English. I didn't know many of the slang words the kids used either.

After the first morning bell, I went to my desk and sat down quietly.

"Can she talk?" one boy, who was sitting in the next row, asked as he pointed at me and looked at the teacher inquiringly.

I died inside, wishing I had been allowed to stay home.

Things got worse at midmorning recess.

"Shut up!" one girl screamed at another one.

"You shut up," the other one screamed back.

"You stupid fool," a boy sneered at another one.

"Hey, what are you looking at, you Greek creep?" one girl shouted at me as I watched the action from the edge of the playground.

Lord, why do I have to come here? I didn't know what bullying was until I came to this school. I remembered how the kids in Athens hugged and kissed me on the last day of school, and I wanted to sob.

The fifteen-minute recess was painfully long.

I went upstairs to my classroom and sat down close to the window. We sat by academic rank. The smartest kids sat by the long side blackboard, the average ones sat in the middle of the class, and the slow ones were seated next to the window. There was no escape from the teacher's judgment; it was plainly visible, and no amount of squirming in your seat would change it.

"Get ready for your arithmetic drills," the teacher snapped. She wound up a kitchen timer and placed it on her desk. "Let's see how fast you can add and subtract now."

Tick, tick, tick, tick, the timer raced quickly.

I was not used to speed tests of any kind and found the pressure terribly unsettling.

"Ding!" The timer rang after ten short minutes.

"Stop!" the teacher said with a sharp tone that matched the timer's bell. Then she quickly walked around the room and picked up our papers.

"All right, now get out your readers," she said in a voice that projected across the room. "Don't just sit there like a bump on a log, get your reader out," she snapped at a boy who seemed to be daydreaming.

The seemingly apathetic boy slowly retrieved his reader from inside his desk.

I dropped my book on the floor as I was trying to get it out of my desk.

"You numbskull!" The teacher was furious. "Pick it up right now, for heaven's sake."

I picked it up as fast as I could, trying not to let the snickers of the other kids bother me, but I felt like a fumbling, incompetent fool. *Everyone is a bully here, even the teacher. And my parents are not happy with my awkward behavior either. Where can I go to feel safe?*

After lunch, the kids went downstairs to the music room to learn musical notation and to sing.

I sneaked away from the group, went back to our empty classroom, and hid under my desk. I didn't have a clue how to read music and was too terrified of having my ignorance exposed.

After a couple of weeks, the music teacher realized what I was doing and gently urged me to come to her class; her soothing tone of voice finally convinced me to go. My ignorance nearly *was* exposed, however, when we had to go up to the blackboard and write the names of the notes under the scale. When it was my turn, I stood with a piece of chalk in my fingers and stared at the meaningless lines with seemingly weird circles and flags. I made a lucky guess and named the note correctly.

My mother was outraged when I told her about my fear of music class and decided it was time for me to take piano lessons.

I loved my piano teacher, who was studying music at the university, and looked forward to Friday afternoons at her house with tremendous anticipation. She told me that music was a mathematical, quantitative art and that people who excelled in it had sophisticated brain power. Someone had told her that she was "just talented" because she was good in music, but she knew that her ability was more than a talent. And when I showed an immediate aptitude for the piano, loved to practice, and advanced quickly, she praised me in a way that greatly boosted my self-esteem. She wrote my homework instructions in a music dictation book, and I would practice as soon as I got home; I was only a few blocks away, and I would rush back to my rented piano.

One of my piano books had a simplified beginner's version of the famous melody of Beethoven's "Ode to Joy," which I played over and over, as if I were possessed by a divine musical energy that was trying to give me a glimpse of heaven on earth. I knew what the great composer was trying to express, and my young soul resonated with the hope of a universal brotherhood. I couldn't understand why some people were cruel and vicious, and I never felt the need to start a fight or hurt anyone on purpose. I would dream about a nonjudgmental world filled with love and acceptance.

In spite of the fact that my parents were sometimes irritated with me, my mother was fiercely protective of me, and my father praised my rational mind and initiated many profound philosophical and scientific discussions with me. We often escaped the city's stresses by driving through the spectacular coastal mountain range to small towns in the interior of British Columbia. Sometimes we hiked in the mountains as well, and the close contact with nature helped me keep things in perspective. This gave me more confidence, and I gradually learned to stand up for myself.

However, the cruelty of some of the kids never ceased to amaze me. One chubby girl was teased so mercilessly for being overweight that her parents were forced to place her in another school; another kid laughed about it and said that she had to "go to a school with wider doors." One boy had a speech impediment that didn't allow him to speak clearly, and he was also teased so relentlessly that he had to leave the school. Another boy had scoliosis, and some kids imitated the way he walked.

Even though I grew stronger, I was still frustrated enough that I would occasionally steal toys from the local drugstore and destroy furniture at home. Some kids found out about this and planned to set a trap for me. A friend told me, "Don't go to that party this weekend. They're planning to put shiny trinkets and jewelry on the table to see if you're going to take them." I was very grateful to her and to anyone else who was honest and kind to me.

I loved Fridays because my piano teacher always treated me with respect. She continued to inspire me, and when I learned to play my first Chopin mazurka, she told me I played it as well as any pianist she had ever heard because I put my heart into the music, as if I completely understood the Polish soul. This boosted my confidence even more. When she returned from a trip to Poland, she gave me a little booklet she had bought in the little town where Chopin was born. I was delighted that she would think of me halfway around the world.

Some of my classmates remained sour, however, even though I excelled academically in junior high. One boy called me a "damn foreigner" because of my long last name, and when I protested and reminded him that I was born in Vancouver and was just as Canadian as he was, he just shrugged and walked away from me without apologizing.

One of my friends knew that my father was born in Smyrna (Izmir), so she attacked me with a vitriolic insult: "You're half-barbarian, and you don't even know it." I was stunned when she told me that the first time, and when she repeated it a little later, I cut her out of my life. By that time, I was more confident about my own inner worth and was convinced that I didn't deserve any of this ignorant nonsense.

Maybe the beauty and hope of the "Ode to Joy" and all it stands for will soften our hearts one day. After all, scientists have recently shown that all humans have very similar DNA, and the differences between us are so slight that we really are all brothers and sisters. We should all be trying harder to love and accept ourselves and others.

Chapter 6

Mother Earth

My grandmother was furious that I had decided to go to a Saturday-evening dance party at Niki's house, but my mind was made up. I asked a friend to drive me there. Niki had given me the address, but I only had a vague idea of where the house was. Luckily for me, my friend had a taxi driver's knowledge of most parts of Athens, and he knew exactly how to get there.

We left the patrician villas and palm-lined streets of my grandmother's suburb and drove toward more modest areas. As we drove, I remembered how kind Niki was to me when I first met her at the age of four. She would often arrive in my grandmother's villa at around 7:00 in the morning and wouldn't leave until she had scrubbed sheets with a washboard in a huge tub, swept floors, scraped scales off fish in the backyard while fending off desperately hungry cats, beat the dust out of rugs hanging on clotheslines, cooked meals, fed the dogs and cats, and cleaned toilets. She consistently worked with great energy and enthusiasm for just a few drachmas.

No matter how busy she was, she was never annoyed with me

when I followed her around the kitchen, the upstairs bedrooms, or the backyard. She often gave me a wide, gap-toothed grin and a hug so huge I felt as if I had been embraced by Mother Earth herself. And when I was sick in bed, she would help my mom take care of me and would sing to me to cheer me up and help me recover.

Soon after I turned fourteen, I returned to Athens for the summer and was stunned when Niki defied my grandmother's gag order and told us that she was my grandmother's first cousin. *Good for you, Niki. You're too poor to be accepted as a relative, but you won't be silenced. Good for you, and now I'm coming to your party.*

"We're almost there," my friend said as we approached a tiny, whitewashed cube of a house that was sitting at the edge of a dusty, weed-infested field. The stark contrast between this area and the wealthy suburb we had left behind was almost obscene. I felt dreadfully sorry for Niki and her family.

"I'll pick you up in a couple of hours," my friend said as I got out of the car.

Niki approached me with open arms and gave me her trademark hug, and her adult kids and their friends also gave me a warm welcome. They led me into the tiny house, which had woven blankets for interior walls and an uneven dirt floor. There were a few naked light bulbs hanging from the ceiling, and there were a couple of narrow mattresses pushed against the outside walls. A little table close to the kitchen area was loaded with dolmades, spanakopita, and tiropita triangles, and I was given a plate and urged to fill it with goodies. Niki told me they had prepared the food with the hope that I would come and enjoy it. I took a sample of each appetizer, and everyone was delighted when they saw how much I enjoyed every morsel.

As soon as I finished, one of my cousins led me outside and asked me to dance. A record player was sitting on a table and was connected to the house with a long extension cord. Another young man announced that he was putting on a bossa nova record. My cousin showed me the dance steps, and then we had a terrific time while everyone else watched. When the second Latin number started, the others joined us, and we danced and laughed with such joy you would have thought we were at the carnival in Rio. When the Greek folk music came on, we danced with that ancient "freedom or die" spirit of resistance against judgment and oppression—the spirit that says, "Hey there, beautiful, don't let the bastards get you down!" I was thrilled to be dancing with my cousins and their friends and even more thrilled that they made such a fuss about me. I was honored to be with such genuine, kind people.

My driver friend arrived a couple of hours later.

"May God always be with you," Niki and her kids told me. "You're such a good soul."

"The same to you," I told them. "Thanks so much for everything."

I learned so much from this visit. I admired Niki for insisting that she be accepted for what she was, and it was clear that she deserved that acceptance. It didn't matter where she lived or what she looked like; she was as hardworking and kind as Mother Earth and deserved to be treated well. Niki and her family did not deserve to be judged and excluded just because they were poor, and I was not ashamed of them. On the contrary, I was proud of their resilient and irrepressible spirits.

Ten years later, I visited Niki again. The government had paid her well for her little cube and her land and built an apartment block where the cube used to be. One of the apartments was free for her, and another was given to her daughter. She could collect some rent as well and no longer had to work for a pittance in someone else's house.

She told me, "God has smiled upon me at last." Niki, which means "victory," was a good name for her.

Chapter 7

Leroy

"I don't want to arrive with thirteen pieces of luggage," my dad said in a grimly determined tone as our train neared the station in St. Louis. "That number follows me wherever I go."

Mom and I grinned at each other and chuckled. "He's a scientist, but he's superstitious."

Dad didn't look amused. "It's not funny! Help me out; there must be something we can do," he said in an agitated tone.

I thought about it for a few seconds. "Oh, I know—the small bag with old books and magazines. I don't really need them anymore, so we can leave that behind on the overhead rack."

Dad nodded, obviously relieved.

We arrived at around 10:00 in the evening of July 4, 1966, and gathered our bags together. The tall, affable black porter walked by the overhead rack, picked up the small, unclaimed bag, and said, "Anybody own this here bag? Anybody?" He picked it up and looked inside. "Books?" He paused. "Okay, then. I guess I'll take it. Might be good for sumpin'," he said in a warm Southern drawl.

No one else said a word, but I was quietly amused by Dad's attempt to control his luck. We actually arrived with thirteen pieces of luggage anyway, even though we left one behind. Thirteen was Dad's lucky number, so I was expecting to have a fascinating year in St. Louis.

We stepped down onto the platform and were nearly knocked flat by the sledgehammer-like humid heat, which was worse than Athens in the summer. We struggled to breathe, and there were no taxis anywhere.

"Excuse me, where are the taxis?" Mom asked the porter in a thin, weak voice.

"There won't be none for a while, Ma'am. It's July 4."

My parents and I gave each other vacant, listless stares. We had forgotten about July 4.

One lone old taxi screeched into the waiting area after about an hour. We were the only people waiting for a taxi in the all-but-deserted station, and we grabbed it. We stayed in a hotel for a few days, and after our furniture arrived from Canada, we moved into a tall brick apartment building that was just a few blocks away from the famous Gaslight Square entertainment district.

Leroy, a short, wiry, older black man whose job was to manage the garage, helped us get settled. He was unusually friendly and very talkative and took us on a tour of the building to see the pool, the different sets of elevators, the laundry room, and other areas. "Anything ah can do for you, you jus' let me know!" He always smiled with childlike innocence and a sparkle in his eye.

I was to start tenth grade in a few weeks, and the nearest high school contacted us and said that I would have to take a "track test" before enrolling. No one explained what that was, and I assumed it would be some sort of sports test.

Early on one lethally hot August morning, I got on a bus and headed for the high school. I didn't feel well enough for any kind of sports test. I had to change buses, and it took almost an hour to get there.

Soon after I arrived in the office, I was led to a dusty, airless classroom and told to sit down and get ready for the test; there were at least twenty other students in the room. The proctor distributed the reading and general knowledge multiple choice tests and told us to sit quietly when we finished them. No directions were given, and I still had no idea why we had to take the test.

The written directions were confusing, and I wasn't sure which sections I was supposed to complete and which sections I was supposed to leave out; some sections were for grade-nine students, others for grade ten, others for grade eleven, and still others for grade twelve. I finished the reading comprehension section quite a bit sooner than the students who were sitting next to me, and I wondered why.

Oh, no, I thought after the whole exam was over. I suddenly realized that I had failed to complete the test, and I had a sick feeling that this would haunt me for a long time to come. I was so upset that I got on the wrong bus and had a devil of a time finding my way back to the apartment.

"What's the matter with you? You look like you seen a ghost," Leroy said to me as I dragged myself toward the garage's entrance.

I told him about the horrible day I had, trying not to cry.

"You gonna be okay, you'll see. Don't you cry, now, you hear? You gonna be okay." He spoke with a very warm, velvety tone.

"Thanks," I muttered. "I'm glad you think so."

He led me to his huge old green Buick and opened up the back trunk, which was overflowing with kitchen utensils, food, and other assorted hardware. "I keep all mah valuables in mah car," he said. He removed the lid of a plastic container and showed me some neat squares of freshly baked cornbread. The soothing aroma wafted up to me and masked the memory of the awful day for a few seconds. "Have some of mah cornbread. I made it this mornin'."

I took a piece out of the container.

"Go on, have a bit. You'll feel better. You too nice to feel bad 'bout nothin'. Go on, take it." He flashed me that happy grin with the dancing eyes.

The cornbread was deliciously warm and moist. After I swallowed a bit, I asked him why he kept his valuables in his car.

"So mah roommates at home won't be stealin' 'em," he said. Then he gave a staccato-like giggle.

I smiled a little until I remembered what a day it had been.

Leroy instantly noticed my involuntary frown. "Keep your chin up. Don't let nothin' get you down."

"Thanks, Leroy. I have to go upstairs now. My parents will be wondering what happened to me." I finished my cornbread, walked slowly toward the nearby elevator, and waved at him.

He waved back with the enthusiasm of a good old buddy.

I went back to the school a few days later to meet with a counselor and to discuss the results of the track test. I climbed several flights of stairs, arrived in the counseling area, and was directed to the office of one of the many counselors; a huge faculty and staff was needed to run the school, which apparently had an enrollment of over two thousand students.

A pleasant-looking middle-aged lady wearing thick glasses looked up at me as I stood before her desk. She confirmed my name, asked me to sit down, and then retrieved a couple of test result papers from the top of a tall inbox pile. I wasn't expecting good news.

"Track two," she said with a curt, matter-of-fact tone. "Yes, we're placing you in track two. Your reading score is kind of low, so we think you can't handle a full course load. Normally you would take biology along with your other subjects, but we strongly recommend that you drop that for this year."

I drew a sharp breath. "But I didn't finish the test because the directions were confusing." I spoke rapidly, hoping she would understand.

She didn't react to what I said; she just insisted that I would be placed in track two.

"How many tracks are there? What is track two?" I could feel the color drain from my face.

"The track-one-A kids are the smartest. They've been accelerated so they'll finish high school a year earlier than the others. The track-one kids are the really good students, the track-two kids are average and sometimes a little below average. The track-three kids are not academically inclined at all. Some of them drop out of school to look for jobs that don't demand much skill." She spoke softly, but she was nonchalant. She obviously had no idea how this rigid judgment and classification was affecting me.

She might as well have told me I did not have a bright future ahead of me. I couldn't believe it. *What will my parents say? What a shame for someone who comes from a family of academics and professionals. What an unspeakable, terrible shame.*

The meeting was over. I kept my head down, rose slowly, and walked back to the stairs. I felt a little dizzy, so I held on to the railing on the way down.

When I arrived back home, Leroy was standing at the entrance of the garage and saw me walking down the street toward him. He waved excitedly. "How you doin'?"

"Not so good," I murmured. Then I explained what had happened.

"Don't you be listenin' to that stuff. You cheer up, now. I can tell by looking at you that you are smart! Never mind what the test says. You are smart, and you gonna prove the teachers wrong." He spoke energetically and stomped his foot down.

"Thanks, Leroy. Nice of you to say so," I said with a downcast look.

"I'm not just being nice. It's true! You wait and see—you'll do so well at school them teachers won't know what to do with you." Leroy's eyes were scintillating.

I managed to give him a wan smile.

I told my mom about the track test fiasco but couldn't bring myself to tell my dad.

By Christmas, I had established myself as one of the best students in the tenth grade. My homeroom teacher was very friendly to me, and I often ran errands for her during study break. My parents suggested I ask her over for dinner one evening, and she came to our apartment with lovely hostess gifts for my mom. She enjoyed our company and the dinner.

In the early spring, my homeroom teacher told me that my marks were so good that the school's computer was a little confused. Track-two students were not supposed to get marks like that.

Once again, I explained the reason for my low reading score on the track test, but she didn't listen any more than the counselor had when she placed me in track two at the beginning of the year.

"You might be able to work your way up to track one if you really try hard—that is, if you stay at this school next year. However, there's no guarantee that you could, and it's out of the question that you'd ever be track-one-A material. Those kids are born sharper than most, and they don't even have to try hard to be accelerated. They're the future leaders of society." She wasn't trying to be mean to me; she just had the unshakeable conviction that she was right. I remembered a joke sign I had seen in a drugstore: "My mind's made up. Don't confuse me with facts." But I didn't feel like laughing.

No matter how hard I tried to dismiss her words about the future leaders of society, I couldn't do it. It was as if she had locked me in a cage with a sign saying, "Average and ordinary, with no potential." She had judged me and categorized me, as if she had the advanced technology to analyze the full capacity of my brain with total accuracy. Even as a baby, I hated being confined in a playpen; the idea of being in a cage was revolting and unacceptable to me.

When I saw Leroy at the garage entrance on Saturday morning, I told him what my homeroom teacher had said and how it made me feel like a caged animal.

"Oh my, oh my." He shook his head. "They never give up trying to judge you, do they? Like what they do to mah people. We been told we got limits over and over again. Hey, it's like we all in track three, with no hope of ever getting out of it."

I laughed, feeling a little better.

"And you know what? We're gonna rise up and prove we're okay. One of these days, we gonna have a black president. And then what will they say?" Leroy cackled like a child.

"I'm so glad you have that free spirit, Leroy. It's always so good to talk to you."

"Remember, God loves all of us. He don't care what track we're in. Don't make no difference to Him." He shook his head. "People are so good at making each other feel bad. Like I told you when I first met you, you too nice for that. And you're too smart and too kind. Forget about them tracks. Just think about God and how much He loves you." He sounded like a preacher who had just seen an angel and paused to watch me reflect on his words. Then he continued in a lighter tone, "You should go to Gaslight Square this evening with your mama and papa. That happy music, it can help you forget about all that stuff that ain't important."

"You're right, Leroy. I'll ask them to take me." I felt even better.

My parents and I had been to the square several times already, and we looked forward to going again.

Soon after we sat down at a table in one of the clubs, a lady from the audience got up on the stage and sang, "You're Nobody Till Somebody Loves You." She sang with passionate joy, and I realized just how true the words were. Love made a mockery out of any kind of judgment.

At the end of June, Dad told me and Mom that he was absolutely thrilled with the results of the heart disease research he had done during the past year in St. Louis. One of his lab assistants, who lived a few blocks away from us, invited us to go to a birthday party at her house. She told Dad we would be the only white people there.

We arrived at the party on a Saturday evening, and the little white-frame house was almost rocking from side to side in time to the music. There were already at least fifty people there, many of them standing around a huge vat in the middle of the kitchen. They beckoned us over to it. "This is the real Kentucky fried chicken," one lady chirped. "You gotta try it."

The vat was filled with chicken pieces floating in an aromatic white sauce. I picked up a piece with a large spoon and placed it on a little plate. One bite was all it took; this was by far the best chicken I had ever tasted. My parents couldn't believe how good it was, either.

As soon as I finished the chicken thigh, a young man led me back to the living room and danced with me. He was so flexible and supple he could have been a circus acrobat. People made room for us and cheered us on.

Everyone in the house was riotously happy, and a brightly decorated cake as long as the dining room table was brought out from the kitchen. When it was cut, my parents and I were given the first pieces. We indeed were the only white people there, but we were treated like guests of honor.

We must be doing something right.

When it was time for us to leave, Dad's lab assistant walked us down the steps and toward the sidewalk. "We're all so happy you could come," she said. "You folks are real special, you know that?"

We grinned at her. "So are you," we said almost at once.

Leroy was waiting for us and was thrilled to hear about the fabulous party and what a fantastic time we had.

He had tears in his eyes a few days later when the moving truck arrived to get our furniture. "Don't you forget what I told you, you hear? I'm gonna miss you and your parents. I know the good Lord wanted us to meet, but it's time to say good-bye for now. We'll meet again."

"Yeah, Leroy, we'll meet again," I said with a thick lump in my throat.

Judging and pigeonholing people by test results that don't measure creativity is almost as damaging as classifying them according to the color of their skin. Psychologists have shown that there are at least twenty-two different types of intelligence, all of them necessary for the smooth functioning of society, and few of them are measured by traditional intelligence and track tests.

Leroy was right to ignore all forms of rigid classification. He was a man of very few material possessions, but he possessed the profound insight that comes from compassion and self-acceptance. And his friendship did wonders for my self-esteem. We're lucky when we meet supportive people like him.

Chapter 8

Desiree

"I know Desiree doesn't care about school, but she knows a lot about history. She's always telling me about ancient Rome or medieval France, and sometimes we even discuss Socrates." I put my fork down and looked at Desiree's father, who was sitting right across from me at the dining room table.

"Oh, please. She just likes the costumes," Desiree's father snorted with amused contempt.

"Now, now, *mon ami*," Desiree's mother said, looking at him with an indulgent smile.

Desiree's brother chortled and squealed as if he had just breathed in the contents of a helium balloon. Then he jumped up and down in his seat.

"Merde," Desiree said as she slapped her brother's arm.

"Well, happy seventeenth birthday to you. You look gorgeous." I raised my wine glass.

"Thanks, kiddo," Desiree said. Her long, brilliant blonde hair was piled up in an elaborate bun and braided with a shiny orange ribbon. Her brown eyes were accented with jungle-green eye shadow, and her tangerine-orange dress matched the ribbon. She was as stunning as Brigitte Bardot.

"That ribbon makes you look like Marcel Marceau," her brother said.

"Shut up, you imbecile," Desiree said, chuckling.

"Happy birthday, thweetie," Desiree's mother said with an affected lisp.

"Hmphh. It was a slip that you were born," her father said with a sly smile.

"It was a case of a slip that wasn't there," Desiree retorted without skipping a beat.

Her mother's face flushed, and her eyes widened with mock surprise.

I chewed a piece of tender chicken cordon bleu to calm my nerves. *What kind of a birthday dinner is this? But why am I surprised? They talk like this to each other most of the time, and Desiree is a preferred target.*

The dinner was so incredibly gourmet, we decided to stop talking to enjoy it.

My mind wandered back to the day I first met Desiree. We were both nine years old. She had just returned to Canada from France, and I had just returned after my two-year stay in Athens. We met one August afternoon at the house of my mom's best friend, and we were so shy we hardly looked at each other as we sat on a big sofa in the living room. The grownups talked and laughed a lot, but we remained silent. When it was time to leave, though, we shook hands and made plans to see each other again.

Desiree soon became my best friend, even though we didn't go to the same school. We had the same sense of humor and enjoyed ourselves even when we just rode our bikes to the corner store. She had seen some of the kids who used to bully me, and she laughed at them.

Just before she turned fourteen, she phoned me. "My mother's sending me away to a boarding school back east. I can't believe it. I wanted to come to your school."

"What? Why?"

"Mom says I'm too rebellious and too difficult to handle."

When Desiree came home for Christmas break, I asked her about school. "I'm having fun," she said. "I get a brainy friend to do my math homework, and I meet my boyfriends in town on weekends. We go dancing, and they fight over me."

Whenever she came home for holidays, she entertained me with stories of her wild escapades, mocking her parents' desperate attempts to control her.

And now, because Desiree refused to stay at the boarding school any longer, she was living at home again, attending my school, and fending off her family's insults at her seventeenth birthday celebration.

After supper, she took me downstairs to the rec room and put a stack of Beatles records in the record player. We danced to "Roll over Beethoven" and other songs.

When we decided to have a break and sit down on the sofa, she lit a cigarette. "You with your good ears—tell me if you hear anyone coming down the stairs," she said. She blew smoke rings toward the ceiling.

"I guess they don't know you smoke," I said.

"Is the pope Catholic? You know how much I love my cigs." She chuckled, and I smiled. "Get ready to wave away the smoke if they come down suddenly."

"Okay," I said. I didn't know what else to do if that happened.

"I can't wait for school to be over." Desiree rolled her eyes. "It's such a waste of time! I'm very ambitious, and I can't wait to get out there and make lots of money. My grandmother still is a really good businesswoman, unlike my intellectual parents, and everyone's always asking her for money. And she's really nice to me too."

"Yes, I still remember that beautiful royal blue velvet skating outfit she bought for you when you were ten," I said. "In fact, she was always buying you clothes."

"Yeah, and she tells me I can move in with her any time. Her new house is just a few blocks down the street." She put out her cigarette in a heavy brass ashtray and waved her arms to dissipate the smoke.

"So are you seriously thinking of moving in with your grandmother?" I lowered my voice.

She nodded. "You know how crazy life is around here." She stared at the rec room door and listened. Not hearing anything, she continued, "Last Sunday I got home at three o'clock in the morning, and my parents were furious. They say they don't understand why I'm so wild."

"Wild? Adventurous and fun-loving, yes, but wild?"

"Yeah, yeah. What else is new?"

Desiree moved in with her grandmother a couple of months later and stayed there until she finished high school.

I took a break from my first year of university studies and went to see Desiree at her grandma's house on one cool Saturday morning. She was standing beside a new electric blue Camaro and wearing a silvery satin blouse, a teal green cummerbund, black leather pants, and black spiked heels. Her long, wavy hair was an iridescent, silvery gold. She smiled at me, not seeming to notice the cars that were cruising slowly down the road in front of the house. The male drivers looked thunderstruck and slack-jawed.

"The way those guys are staring—that's just too funny," I said as I shook my head.

"Oh? Oh yeah, those guys. That happens all the time. I don't pay any attention to them." She opened the passenger door. "Do you wanna go to Chinatown for lunch?"

"Sure!" I hopped in the car.

We took off with a terrific roar. "Like the car?"

I nodded. "Where did you get it?"

"One of my business partners is lending it to me for as long as I want it," she said.

"Business partners?"

"Yeah. I've met some guys who are as business-minded as I am. We've teamed up and formed our own salvaging company, and we're into buying real estate. I love being around people who have that enterprising spirit. I just love it!" She changed lanes and passed yet another thunderstruck man who turned his head to gape at her.

"That guy has really round, sleepy blue eyes," I said as I smirked.

"We'll call him *halibut*," she said. Then she sped up so much I gripped the dashboard.

"Look behind us—are there any cops following us?" she asked as she kept speeding.

"No, but I don't think they'd be able to catch up with us anyway," I said.

We made it to Chinatown in record time, passing red and gold street signs with Chinese characters and a martial arts school. "That's where I'm learning kung fu," Desiree said. She pointed to the second floor of the building. "My teacher is eighty-five years old!"

"What?" I asked, laughing.

"Hey, you should see him in action. He's a wiry little guy from Hong Kong, and he often asks three young guys to attack him at once. No matter how hard they try to do him in, he knocks them flat in seconds. Seconds! He's the best teacher in town."

We parked beside a red telephone booth that looked like a pagoda. "See that bank behind the telephone booth?"

"Yeah."

"A white guy tried to hold it up a few days ago. He gave the Chinese teller a hold-up note written in English. She didn't understand the note, so she showed it to the manager, and he didn't understand it either. They talked so fast and loud in Chinese that it scared the guy so much he ran out of the bank. The police caught him a few minutes later."

"You sure feel at home here, even though you don't know Chinese," I said.

"Sure do," she said.

I admired her sense of adventure and curiosity about the world.

We walked into a small restaurant across from the bank and sat down at a round table next to a beautiful jade elephant and a potted plant. Soon after the waiter took our drink order, a smartly dressed young Chinese man waved at Desiree from across the room and walked toward us. She waved back and said, "That's one of my business partners."

He sat down, and Desiree introduced us. "By the way, lunch is on me," he said.

"No, no," I said.

"Oh, yes. Don't worry about it," he said.

We enjoyed a seafood hotpot, chicken in paper with brown spices, a Buddha's feast, and rice.

"That was the best Chinese food I've ever had," I said. "Thanks so much."

The business partner produced a long envelope and gave it to Desiree. "Round trip to Hong Kong. You're leaving in two weeks, and our investors will meet you at the hotel. You're tough and smart enough to handle them."

Desiree grinned. "I can't wait. I love a challenge."

What an incredible life she's made for herself. But it isn't good enough for her parents.

Desiree drove me home just in time for supper.

My mother was furious. "Where have you been? That Desiree is a bad influence on you. You could have spent the afternoon studying instead of wandering around with her. How do you think she got that fancy car and those flashy clothes?"

"I don't know that, but I do know that she has a head for business and she's really nice to me. And how come you always touch her hair and tell her how beautiful she is and that you used to look like her when you were younger? How come?" My voice was strident.

Mother just glared at me. "Supper's ready, and your dad can't wait any longer."

I was furious. Desiree was always supportive, encouraging me to visualize myself as free, happy, and successful. She didn't understand why my parents were so strict and didn't want me to wear cute clothes, wear any makeup, or curl my hair.

A week later, after supper, Desiree and I went dancing at a fancy club in the Italian section of town. We sat at a booth next to the dance floor and watched the strobe light send colored rays through the rising dry ice fog. A couple of young guys sat down and tried to talk to us, but the music was a little too loud to have a meaningful conversation.

When the music stopped, Desiree introduced the two men. They were apparently the owners of the club. An older lady walked toward us. "That's Mother. She takes care of the books," they said.

A waitress appeared with a drink tray. "Have a Kahlua and cream," one of the men said. "It's on the house."

"Thanks," I said. Desiree and I sipped our drinks and smiled at each other as the mother sat down with us.

As soon as the music started, we all got up to dance.

We stayed for a couple of hours, and then the two men accompanied us to the door. I stepped into the well-lit parking lot and then looked back to see where Desiree was. One of the men grabbed her and tried to kiss her, but she managed to break away.

"Let's go to the espresso bar down the street for a nightcap," she said as she approached me.

When we arrived, four men jumped up from their seats and ran to greet Desiree. A fifth man, overwhelmed by her beauty, stood trembling by the cash register and with quivering lips, whispered, "Ciao, Bella!" Desiree didn't even notice him.

The lights were very low, and all the tables had the traditional red-and-white checkered tablecloths and chianti bottles smothered with candle wax. A chubby young boy wearing heavy black shoes and white bobby socks was playing "O Sole Mio" on his accordion. He didn't look happy and wanted to stop, but the men coaxed him to keep playing. It was obvious they would do anything to keep Desiree amused for as long as possible. After a coffee and a tiramisu, we headed to the door. "Ciao, Bellissima," the fifth man said in a hoarse voice, once again overwhelmed and ignored.

When we stopped at an intersection before going up a steep hill, a car pulled up beside us. A man with large, round blue eyes gaped and smiled at Desiree. "Hey, there's *halibut* again," we exclaimed at the same time. We left him far behind and laughed all the way home.

A couple of days later, my mother told me that she had heard from Desiree's grandmother about our espresso bar visit. "You need to be more careful. Don't you know that the men in those bars put drugs into the coffee to knock you out so they can rape you? I'm telling you again, that Desiree is a daredevil. She's a bad influence, and your father agrees with me." She scolded me as if I were a clueless five-year-old.

"And I'm telling you again that she may be a daredevil, but she's smart and ambitious. She's nice to me and believes in me. And she doesn't expect me to copy her lifestyle. She knows I'm my own person, and she respects that," I said in a resolute tone.

Mother had no answer.

Desiree loved Hong Kong. She showed me lots of pictures of the city and her hotel. I was particularly impressed with one picture. In it she was standing by a screen and giving a presentation about Vancouver's Chinatown to several smartly dressed men in an executive boardroom. I was really happy for her and admired her determination to succeed.

When I saw her a couple of weeks later, she seemed to be ecstatic. "Guess what?"

"You're going to start your own business without any partners," I said.

"No! Much better than that!"

"Really?"

"I'm going to Paris! Paris! I'm so excited I could fly to Venus and back. I've saved up enough money to live there comfortably for at least a year."

"How long are you going for?"

"I'm moving there permanently. I'm too bored around here, and I'm sick and tired of all the criticism. My parents are always comparing me to all those girls who go to university. I don't need to go there. You know how I've always loved books." She showed me Jean-Paul Sartre's *Huis Clos*.

"Oh, I've read some Sartre. He said, 'Hell is other people.' It's the concept of the horizontal hell. It's right here because of the way we treat each other," I said.

"But Paris will be a step above this little hell. It has to be," she said.

"I'll really miss you, but I understand your need to go there."

"I would have been so much better off with a mother like yours," she said as she put out her cigarette. "Yours is there when you need her. She's a very conscientious mother."

"I know. She's a character, and she's sometimes too tough, but she's there for me."

We laughed. Then she poured us a little Grand Marnier, and we sipped it slowly and quietly.

"Wow, that's good," I said. "Mmmm. To your new life," I said as I raised my glass.

Desiree gave me a pile of fabulous, almost brand new clothes just before she left for Paris.

"Are you sure you don't need these anymore?" She was always generous, but this was amazing.

"Nope, don't need them. I get bored with clothes really fast."

"Thanks, and write soon," I said.

"I'll call you after I'm settled in an apartment."

We hugged, and I took off with the clothes.

Desiree called me after she found an apartment in Paris and told me she was working for a prominent businessman. She had to work very hard, but she was thrilled to be living there.

She came home a year later for Christmas, dressed like a model and full of enthusiasm for her new life. She was more generous than ever, offering me an all-expenses-paid trip to France.

I went to Athens in the summer after I finished my undergraduate degrees in English and music. My uncle met me at the airport in the brilliantly hot afternoon and drove me to my grandmother's villa. He couldn't get over the fact that I wasn't planning to study medicine. My grandmother was one of the first women in Athens to set foot in a medical school, and she was so proud of that she never let anyone forget it. I was expected to follow in her footsteps, and she had brainwashed my uncle to think the same way.

When we arrived at the villa, I was stunned to see that my grandmother was totally blind. I sat down beside her on a sofa in the big living room and greeted her. Instead of greeting me, she groped at my arms and told me I was a failure and that I had to do something much greater with my life.

I had just arrived, but I couldn't wait to leave and go to Paris to visit Desiree. I kept looking at my plane ticket to make sure I only had to stay in Athens for ten days.

Those ten days felt like two months.

Desiree met me at the airport in the afternoon, and we took a taxi to her apartment, which was in Passy, a very pleasant suburb in the sixteenth arrondissement. I had an intense feeling of déjà vu as we drove past some of the famous landmarks. *Of course, this feels so familiar. Dad and I broke up our Athens-to-Vancouver trip and stayed here for two days when I was nine years old. He took me to the Louvre and the second floor of the Eiffel Tower, and we had lunch on the Champs-Elysées. I had a mushroom omelet. Desiree must have been to the same places, and then I met her a couple of months later on another continent. I'm so happy to be far away from my disapproving relatives.*

"What are you thinking? You look like you're so far away," Desiree said as we passed a lovely flower market.

"I'm just reminiscing about the time my dad brought me here. It's a very warm feeling, especially because you might have been here at the same time as I was before I met you. You have no idea how glad I am to be here!" I told her about my unpleasant stay with my relatives.

"Forget about your grandmother. People *like* you, and you're smart and talented. Don't let anyone get you down like that. You don't deserve it." She sounded so affectionate that it eased my painful feelings of rejection.

"Sorry to talk about depressing things like that. I won't any more. Thanks for the support."

"Anytime. What are good friends for?" she said, grinning at me.

We arrived at her relatively modern apartment block, took the elevator to the third floor, and stopped in front of a large, polished wood door with a brassy trim.

"It's almost impossible to find an apartment in this city," Desiree said as she fished out her keys from a large leather purse. "I had to wait for someone to die before I could move in here."

We walked in to a very spacious, airy apartment with a large living room and kitchen, several bedrooms, and a long veranda overlooking the street. One long living room wall was lined with stacks of books. "I'm still waiting for some of my furniture to be delivered, but at least I have my books," she said. "I hope you don't mind," she said.

"Mind?" I laughed. "Who cares about lots of furniture? We're in Paris."

She laughed too.

The doorbell rang. "That's probably the concierge," Desiree said.

"*Voila, mademoiselle,*" a lady said as she presented Desiree with an enormous bouquet of mixed flowers.

"*Merci,*" Desiree replied as she took the flowers. "These are going on the veranda, next to my rose bushes."

"Who sent them? Do you know?"

"A businessman I met last week. I get flowers all the time," she said as she walked toward the veranda. She placed the flowers on a little table, and we sat outside.

"I can sure feel the jet lag now," I said as I sniffed the flowers.

"I believe it," she said. "We'll wait a couple of days before I take you to my office."

Desiree cooked a wonderful ratatouille Provençale and filet mignon for our supper.

A couple of days later, in the middle of a very hot July morning, she took me to her office, which was on the second floor of a beautiful, classically ornate building not too far from the Arc de Triomphe. It was furnished with elegant antiques and had a plush, dark red rug that matched the wallpaper. Her boss, who wasn't in yet, had an even larger and more impressive office, and there were several other offices in the same suite.

"How do you like my office?" Desiree asked as she sat down at her carved desk.

"This is amazing," I said as I sat on an ultra-comfortable chair. "I … I knew it would be impressive, but this is much more than I expected." I was in awe as I looked around the room.

"I'm glad you like it. I do too, of course. I'm in seventeenth heaven here. My boss is fantastic, and so are all the other people I work with." I had never seen her so happy and so radiant.

After she checked her telex messages, she took me around the suite to meet her coworkers, who were all cheerful and very polite. They beamed when I greeted them in French.

Then the elevator door opened, and a man with a booming, commanding voice approached us. His stride was quick, and his eyes were sparkling. "That's my boss," Desiree whispered.

"Bonjour, bonjour," he said to everyone. He nodded at Desiree and shook my hand with a powerful, masculine grip. I loved that.

I spoke a little French with him, and then he told Desiree he would take us out for lunch in a couple of hours.

I kept Desiree company as she took care of some paperwork in her office. "I'm so happy you're here," she said. "I wish you could visit more often."

"How did you get to work in a fabulous place like this?"

"When I first came to Paris, I taught English privately. My boss speaks German really well, but he also wanted to learn English. I saw an ad in the paper, and it led me to this office. After I gave him a few lessons, he realized I loved the business world more than anything else, so he offered me a job as an assistant in the commodities department of his company. One thing led to another, and here I am. I always had the feeling I'd get a great job like this, even before I left Vancouver."

"Well, congratulations. I'm really proud of you," I said.

"Thanks. I wish my dad would think the same way. He visited me a few months ago and told me the Parisians would never fully accept me because I grew up in Canada and my French accent would never be authentically Parisian. What a rotten thing to say. I refuse to speak to him until he apologizes."

"How ridiculous. Your French is perfect. You were bilingual before you could walk."

"I know." Desiree rolled her eyes and curled her lip.

Desiree's boss took us out for lunch at a traditional French restaurant close to the office. We sat at a small, round table, and her boss asked me lots of questions about my life. He spoke French so quickly I didn't always understand him, so Desiree translated for us.

"Where's the salad? Are they still waiting for the lettuce to grow and the tomatoes to ripen?" He pretended to be very impatient when the waiter appeared by his side. "Where's the wine? Are you still squashing the grapes?" He gave the waiter a disarming smile.

I laughed, and he winked at me. *He's winking at me, and I'm not even a beauty queen like Desiree. Very interesting. He's middle-aged, and I'm still young. I guess he likes my innocence. Maybe he even likes my character.*

The waiter eventually did bring the wine, the salad, and the rest of the courses. After the boss paid for our fabulous lunch, he said he would fly us down to Nice for a few days.

"He owns a bicycle factory down there, among other things," Desiree said. "He owns enterprises all over the world, and one of my jobs is to help with advertising the products."

"But I don't have extra money for a trip to Nice," I said.

Desiree told her boss, and he said money was no object and that it was his pleasure to pay for me as well.

"Merci, beaucoup, monsieur. Votre generosite est incroyable," I said.

"C'est rien," he replied.

"I have to go back to the office, but you can spend the rest of the afternoon sightseeing. I'll meet you at the front door of the office around six. You'll be able to find your way back there, won't you?" she asked, looking hopeful.

"Of course, I'll be fine, and I'll see you later," I said.

A couple of days later, Desiree's boss and his chauffeur arrived at the apartment in a late-model black Citroen. Desiree and I got in the backseat, and we were off to the airport. The morning traffic was very heavy, and the boss quickly got impatient with the chauffeur's overly careful driving. "I'm going to drive the rest of the way," he snapped. We stopped for a few seconds so the men could exchange places. The boss drove as if he were on a wide racetrack, careening in and out of lanes constantly. I got a glimpse of his triumphant smile as I glanced at the rearview mirror.

We just made the airbus flight to Nice and arrived in the Cote d'Azur in the early afternoon.

"Feel that silky air, and look at those lovely palm trees," I said. "I love it already."

"I know, I wish I could move down here," Desiree said to me while her boss waved at a nearby taxi. "I like Paris, but Nice has a much warmer climate. My boss prefers Paris, though." She gave a little sigh of resignation.

We stopped at a modern hotel. "Here we are. Your room has already been paid for. Just tell them your name at the reception desk and get your key. I'll come get you in a little while, and we can go exploring," Desiree said.

We strolled around the old town and the Promenade des Anglais all afternoon and admired the dreamy blue sea, the colorful Franco-Italian architecture, and the fabulous shops.

"After we get back to the hotel, you can freshen up. Then I'll come to your room and we'll meet my boss in the lobby so we can go for dinner," she chirped in an upbeat tone.

"I can't wait," I said.

Desiree and I went to the hotel lobby in the evening and joined her boss and another distinguished-looking gentleman and his wife. "This is one of my boss's business partners," Desiree said as she introduced us. They both appeared to be genuinely happy to meet me.

"Vous etes tres jolie," Desiree's boss said to me. *"Tres, tres jolie."* When he kissed me on the cheek, I felt a warm, tingling sensation all over.

We got in a taxi and soon arrived at an exclusive restaurant. The waiter invited us to have predinner drinks on the patio while waiting for our inside table to be ready.

"A votre sante," I said to the group as I lifted my glass of red wine.

Desiree's boss lifted his glass directly to me and said, "I will marry you."

I was speechless, and Desiree drew a sharp breath. "But your wife just passed away last year," she said with a barely audible voice.

"That doesn't matter," Desiree's boss said energetically.

"What about your three kids? What would they think about this?" Desiree went pale.

I laughed, and then everyone except Desiree laughed too.

"You like to joke, *n'est-ce pas?*" I said as I nodded at Desiree's boss.

"Ah, *oui*," he said with an unwavering gaze.

We went inside for dinner and feasted on scampi, chateaubriand, champagne, and countless other delicacies. *Was he just joking, or is he really attracted to me?*

After dinner, we all strolled on the vibrant Promenade des Anglais. Desiree told me there were business meetings the next morning and that she would contact me when they were over.

The next afternoon, the business partner's wife picked Desiree and me up with her Peugeot and drove us to Cannes and Monaco. No matter how spectacular the scenery was, Desiree didn't talk much.

"The wife doesn't speak English, so I can talk about this," Desiree said on the way back to Nice.

"I really envy my boss's wonderful family life. He's such a good father. One of his daughters is a real brain and is studying to become a surgeon. He's very supportive of her. He gave everything to those kids, including private academic and sports lessons. They have a city house and vacation cottages. His son wants to learn the family business, and my boss is teaching him a lot. I can't even imagine what it would have been like to grow up like that." She sounded forlorn.

"I can't either. That total support just isn't there for us, but you're making the best of it. Look how far you've come, working for a man like that. You certainly are a useful employee for him," I said in an optimistic tone.

"Yeah, you're right, but I envy his kids." She sighed. "I would have been much more educated, accomplished, and confident with a father like that."

The three of us had to return to Paris a couple of days later. Desiree's boss whispered in her ear as we walked toward the gate at the Nice airport, and then she speeded up and walked ahead of us. "I enjoy your company very much," he said when she was out of earshot.

"Thank you," I said softly.

"I would like to help you get a job in Nice." I was simultaneously flattered, overwhelmed, scared, excited, thrilled, and stunned. There were even some emotions I had never felt before. I admired him, but I had no idea what to say. We didn't break our stride as we continued toward the gate.

I cleared my throat. "How generous and thoughtful of you. I'll have to think about it, and I'll let you know my decision soon. I have to fly back to Canada in a few days." I spoke in an even tone, hoping to control my emotions.

"*Bien sur!*" He nodded and we caught up with Desiree at the gate soon after that.

The chauffeur was waiting for us with the black Citroen when we got back to the Paris airport, and he drove us back to Desiree's apartment. "*Au revoir*, and think about the offer," Desiree's boss told me when we got out of the car. Desiree looked perplexed and worried but said nothing.

I smiled at her boss and thanked him profusely for the fabulous trip to Nice.

"See you at work," Desiree's boss told her just before he and his chauffeur sped away.

"What was that all about?" Desiree asked after we got back into her apartment.

"Your boss must be convinced that I also want to live in France. He's offered to help me get a job in Nice," I said with a steady voice.

Desiree did not reply. She lit a cigarette, poured herself a big glass of Beaujolais, walked out to the veranda, and sat down. She was obviously too preoccupied to ask me if I wanted wine, so I helped myself and joined her out on the veranda.

"It doesn't bother you to smoke and drink at the same time? I tried that once, and it made me sick," I said, wincing.

"Nah. I've been smoking for years, and I won't stop because my cigs calm me down."

Desiree and I had similar problems. She had made a physical escape from her judgmental parents, but she needed to make an internal escape by learning to accept herself totally. She was halfway around the world, but those pernicious voices were still living in her mind. Her glamor didn't have the power to silence them. She was probably romantically attracted to her boss because he represented the kind of loving father she didn't have. It was not surprising that she couldn't stop smoking.

My own youthful days would have been infinitely easier if I would have been able to accept myself at that time. Maybe I would have been able to sit in the plane and laugh all the way from Athens to Paris instead of complaining about my family to Desiree.

Chapter 9

The Rocket Scientist

"One day we'll have the technology to make the earth itself into a rocket ship, and we'll be able to travel to other stars without leaving home. I enjoy playing with my dog in the backyard too much, and I can't imagine putting myself or anyone else through all that rigorous training for space travel."

I could always count on hearing something wondrous and inspiring whenever I went to visit our family friend the rocket scientist. He had published several scientific research papers and was often invited to speak at international space program conventions. When he was younger, he travelled all over the United States to give lectures and to help the Americans catch up with the Soviets after they launched Sputnik.

"When I was at the last convention a couple of months ago, a scientist asked me what religion I was." Our friend chuckled and shook his head. "With a very straight face, I told him I was an Intergalactic Redemptionist. He never got it." His eyes were alive with a mischievous twinkle.

He was always brilliant and humorous when I was visiting for dinner.

I was amazed that he was not in the least bit chauvinistic. "Women should be running the world, no question about it," he said with an authoritative tone of voice.

"Really? Why?" I gazed at him with intense curiosity.

"Because they know how to run a household, and they know how to apply the same principles when they're in government positions. They know how to manage, and they don't waste valuable energy in useless ego fights."

"It's amazing that you would think that," I said. "Many women don't believe in themselves as much as that. They should listen to you."

He grinned. "And women have proven themselves in the hard sciences as well. In fact, I just read about a young woman in Russia who figured out a 'moments of inertia' problem that was supposed to have been unsolvable."

"Thanks for telling me that! I'll remember all this the next time I meet a chauvinist." It did wonders for my female psyche to hear such a brainiac defend my sex.

"My pleasure," he said. "I always enjoy talking to you because you're always smiling."

He picked up a picture from a shelf behind the dining room table. "I want to show you a picture of my brother," he said.

He placed it before me. I shrieked with laughter when I saw the large, clear photo of an enormous silverback gorilla surrounded by bright green jungle foliage.

"I can't wait to show this to my grandchildren when they come over tomorrow," he said.

After dinner one evening, he showed me some of his recently published papers. They were unwieldy in their complexity. "Wow," I whispered. "Imagine having the intellect to do this."

He sighed long and hard. "Yes, but I'm not as smart as some of those others who get prizes."

I felt so sorry for him that I was speechless. Many people all over the world would have given away their firstborn child to have his intellect, notoriety, and achievements. Rocket science is popularly described as one of the hardest, most exclusive disciplines of our time, reserved only for those few who are at the very far end of the intelligence spectrum.

When a rocket scientist judges himself to be inferior to other scientists, you just know that we humans have created a horizontal hell for ourselves. What logical answer can you give when you keep asking, "Why?" *Why should I feel inferior because I didn't get a prize?*

Chapter 10

Venus

I always looked forward to my university art class, which was held twice a week after lunch. I headed toward a front-row desk, sat down, retrieved a notebook from my briefcase, and perused my notes from the previous class while my fellow students rushed into the small classroom and got settled.

Pete, a talented graphic artist who usually sat quite far away from me, suddenly appeared right next to me.

"Hi! You don't mind if I sit beside you, do you?" His voice was unctuous.

"No. Why should I mind?" I gave him a half smile.

"Good." He produced a notebook and began drawing a humpback whale with a blue pencil.

As I watched him draw, my eyes widened. In just two or three minutes, a beautiful whale appeared on just half a sheet of paper. "It's amazing how you can do that so fast," I said.

"I've always loved art," he said cheerfully as he drew waves around the whale.

The professor sauntered in and started setting up a slide projector. At the speed he was going, it was obvious we'd have some more time to talk.

Pete leaned down, grabbed an art history book out of his satchel, and opened it up to the Italian renaissance section. "May I put this on your desk? You'll see the pictures better that way."

"Sure," I said.

"I love these paintings," he said as he slowly turned the pages.

"I do too. They're beautiful, yes, but they honor the human soul and spirit. They're celebrating life itself." There were many paintings I had never seen before.

Then he turned a page and stopped at Botticelli's *Birth of Venus*. I drew a sharp breath.

We both stared at the magnificent painting as if we had unearthed a long-lost treasure.

"That's you," Pete said casually, pointing to Venus.

I was speechless. *He must be joking.*

"I've been meaning to sit beside you ever since this class started, but I finally worked up the nerve today. I've admired you for months. You look like a Renaissance painting, and you're a multitalented Renaissance woman as well."

"Th … thanks … but … you hardly know me," I said quietly.

"Oh, I know you. Your looks tell me everything." He spoke with unflappable confidence.

The professor got his projector working, so we had to pay attention to him, but I couldn't stop thinking about Pete's confession.

After class, Pete and I strolled around the campus. He told me he was living with a very nice woman but that he wanted to be my friend.

I wondered what he really meant by *friend. He tells me I look like Venus and he just wants to be friends? Hmmm.*

"You always wear such bright, colorful clothes," Pete said jauntily.

"Thanks. It's reverse psychology. If you wear bright colors, you feel bright," I said.

"Not like me. I'm always in drab colors, usually gray, as I'm sure you've seen." He gave me a self-deprecating grin.

I laughed, feeling a little more at ease with him.

He pointed to his well-worn gray runners. "Even these are gray, like the weather."

We walked over a grassy area close to the imposing Gothic library. "Just think how hard the gardeners have to work to keep up these grounds," I said.

"Yes, and tell me, do you think those scholars whose books are in that library are superior to the gardeners? Is their work more valuable for mankind than the work of the guy who mows the grass?" He made a sweeping gesture with his arm, as if to show the vastness of the lawn.

"It depends on the type of scholar. A scientist who finds a cure for a disease and helps millions of people would be invaluable. Of course that work would be superior to that of the gardener," I said in a firm tone.

"But the gardener's work brings great joy to the whole campus. Is that really inferior to anything or anyone?"

"But does it help as many people?" I arched an eyebrow.

"Maybe it does. How do we really know for sure? Is there a way we could actually prove who is better for mankind?" he asked in a challenging tone.

"Well, it would be hard to actually prove, but we've come a long way in the last few thousand years because of those scholars."

"The gardeners, and people like them, might have made it possible for the scholars to concentrate on their work, so the gardeners' work would be just as valuable. It is just like a good housewife who makes it possible for a man to excel in his work." He gave me a triumphant smile, knowing that he had made an unassailable point. "And maybe the beauty the gardener creates is the greatest inspiration of all."

"It's all food for thought, I must admit." I nodded slowly. *He sure has intellectual depth, persistence, and tenacity.*

We continued walking and arrived in the plush residential area adjacent to the campus. Many of the dwellings were mansions, and a couple looked like castles. I lived several blocks away, in a more modest section of the area.

"God, it's quiet here. There's not a soul anywhere. All these mansions, all this wealth and status, and yet there is no soul. Brrrrr!" Pete shivered and stopped walking to gaze at the houses.

"You're right," I said. I was amazed that he could assess the place so quickly and so accurately. I was so used to the ambience that I had suppressed my awareness of it.

"I live in a working-class neighborhood, and I wouldn't live anywhere else. It has warmth and soul. People are outside talking and laughing, and you see cats and dogs chasing each other."

I looked at my watch. "I have to go to my next class now, so we better head back."

"Yeah, I have a class too," he said.

In the spring, close to the end of the academic year, Pete and I walked to a rose garden that overlooked the ocean. We sat down on a stone bench and admired the afternoon view.

"You look even lovelier than you did before Christmas," Pete said as he looked me up and down. "Your eyes have more depth, and you look even more confident. And your light pink and robin's egg blue clothes bring out the freshness of your spirit." He looked directly into my eyes, as if trying to examine my brain.

"Thanks. And I see you've still got your usual, comfortable clothes," I said.

He laughed. "Yup, still the same old gray and the same old runners. Love 'em."

I gazed at the ocean and the mountains and sighed.

"You want to accomplish a lot in life, but you're not quite sure what it is yet." He spoke in a friendly brotherly tone, but his eyes were still trying to penetrate my mind.

"That's true. I keep dreaming and hoping." I nodded and smiled.

"You have more than it takes to succeed. You've got strength, brains, and looks."

"Oh, you and your exaggerations," I said, smirking.

"I'm not exaggerating. In fact, if you were a man and had all the same qualities, I'd want to kill you."

My jaw dropped.

"But since you're a woman, I figure you'll be frustrated enough in your life, so I won't wish you any extra harm." He gave me a sunny, toothy grin.

"How kind of you." I curled my lip and turned my head away. *He may be profoundly intelligent, but his heart seems to be ruled by insecurity and irrational jealousy.*

Chapter 11

Charles

Charles grabbed me and kissed me on the mouth with such force I could hardly breathe. He had the tenacity of a pit bull and wouldn't let go of me no matter how hard I tried to pull away from him.

When I finally did break away, I rushed out to his fifth-floor balcony and stared at the simmering violet and apricot sunset to try to calm myself. *What am I going to do now?* Charles was tall and muscular and was used to getting his own way because he was an established professor of music and a well-known concert pianist.

Charles followed and put his arm around me. "Will you marry me?"

This is insane. It's only a first date, and he's twenty-five years older than I am.

"Well? What do you say? You won't find anyone with a better profession." He looked perfectly smug. "And I also think we'd make beautiful love together."

"I don't know what to say. I've never been proposed to before,"

I said. "And this is so … so sudden. We hardly know each other. Okay, you were one of my professors a few years ago, but that's all it was. You gave us your lectures and your exams, and that was it. There was nothing personal."

"I proposed to my wife on our first date, and the marriage lasted for thirty years. We've just divorced, but we're still friends, so I'm obviously an excellent judge of character. What do you say to that?" Charles grinned like a boxer who had just flattened his opponent after only thirty seconds in the ring.

"I … I say I don't know you well enough to give you an answer. You're … very handsome and I'm very attracted to you, but you're so much older than I am. I hope to marry someone closer to my own age." *Why, oh, why did I agree to come to his apartment after dinner?* I realized that I should have insisted on going back to my own place.

"I was stunned by your beauty when I picked you up tonight. I nearly fell backward on your landlady's stairs when I saw you." Charles whistled like a teenager, and I giggled. "Come here, you gorgeous thing." He hugged me and kissed every part of my face.

When I pulled back a little, Charles became very agitated.

"Come on, let's go!" His voice was deep as he tilted his head in the direction of the bedroom.

"No! No!" *All I need now is to get pregnant.* My parents had made it very clear that they would not support me if I got pregnant without being married. I couldn't afford to let this happen and watch my dreams for the future crash into a garbage dump.

"What are you scared of? Let's go! Now!" Charles finally overpowered me and pulled me into his bedroom.

"I'm not used to this," I said. "I've been out with lots of guys, but it never got this far."

"I love you!" Charles didn't seem to hear what I was trying to say. "You love me, don't you? I think you do."

"I'm attracted, but I don't know about love. I really should go home now," I said in a raspy voice.

"I love you too much to let you go, and I need you," he said in a stubbornly desperate tone.

*****

"I'm going to have a shower, and then I'm going to make breakfast," Charles said at just after 7:00 in the morning. He leaned over in the bed and kissed me. "You look even more beautiful now, my love. You know I love you." He tried to sound very convincing.

I didn't feel beautiful. I felt horrible, and I wondered what I was doing in that strange bedroom.

Charles did everything in a tremendous hurry. He was dressed and already making breakfast while I walked toward the bathroom.

I sat down at the little bridge table and sipped the hazelnut-flavored coffee he had placed before me. He removed some toast and Pop Tarts from the toaster oven and some hard-boiled eggs from the fridge. "I'm trying to get used to living alone and cooking for myself," he said. "And I hope you don't mind the bridge table. I needed something in a hurry, but I'll get better things soon. The upright piano over there has a mute, which is good when you're in an apartment. My grand is in storage."

"Was your wife a good cook?"

"When she felt like it, yes, but she prefers improving her mind. She's a brilliant woman with a huge vocabulary, and she even started writing a novel a few years ago." He placed the food on the table and then opened the fridge to look for butter.

"How far is she with her novel?" I chewed a piece of dry brown toast.

"I don't think she'll ever finish it. She gets these obsessions, but she can't follow through." Charles smiled at me, leaned over the table, and kissed my cheek. "But you're going to follow through with whatever you do."

"I will? That's good to know." I was grateful for his compliment, but I felt a bit sorry for his wife. "By the way, why did you divorce if you were married so long and you still admire her intelligence so much?"

"We clashed too much during the last few years. Also, I think she's become a lesbian." Charles sat down, had a sip of coffee, and munched on a strawberry Pop Tart.

I was hoping to escape soon, and I looked toward the window. "The sun's coming out. That's great because I have lots of errands to do today, and I'm meeting some friends later on." I spoke in an urgent tone, trying to make him understand that I really did have other things to do.

Charles suddenly fanned his fingers out with a flamboyant gesture and stared at them.

I was struck by the great size of his hands. "Your hands remind me of Artur Rubinstein's. I remember seeing a picture of them on the cover of *Time* magazine."

"Thank you, honey. Stay with me today. Do you really have to go out? I need you." He scrutinized his hands and moved his fingers as if he were playing a keyboard.

"Yes, I have to go," I said with a strong voice. I was very anxious to leave, no matter how much he told me he loved me and needed me.

"Move in with me, honey. If I had you by my side, I'd feel like playing again. There are some new pianists in town, and some people say they're better than I am, but when I'm with you, I'm on top of the world. I need you." Charles was whining like a little boy.

"Who cares about those other pianists? Everyone knows how good you are." I frowned.

"I had to work very hard to get where I am and didn't have time to really enjoy life. The others didn't have to work as hard as I did to reach the same level." He looked pitiful.

"How do you know for sure they didn't have to work as hard? And even if they didn't have to, so what? Look where you are now. You've made it. Isn't that what counts?" I didn't like his negative, highly competitive attitude. It was depressing to listen to him, and I couldn't wait to get out in the sun and the fresh air to shake off the oppressive feeling of frustrated ambition. Several of the professors I met at that time were like him. No matter how accomplished they were, they were never satisfied, and they couldn't find peace or happiness. They also were impatient with those who were not as driven as they were.

Charles and I dated for a few weeks and went to some of the best restaurants in the city for gourmet dinners. He kept insisting that I move in with him and marry him, and I kept insisting that I loved him but couldn't marry him because he was so much older and I eventually wanted to start a family. A suffocating feeling of hopeless impasse hung over us wherever we went.

Charles picked me up one clear morning and drove me to the marina where his motor boat was docked. We jumped in the boat and took off to explore hidden inlets and small islands. The boat was comfortable, so I could relax and absorb the mysterious beauty of the coast.

"You look like you're enjoying yourself," Charles said when we reached a shallow cove.

"I love it. I've always loved nature," I said. I closed my eyes and breathed in the marine air, which was saturated with the smells of kelp, algae, salty fish, and motor oil.

"You remind me of an innocent young fawn," he said. "You have those big, placid eyes and that gentle nature. In fact, you're too gentle. Nice guys finish last in this world."

I flinched. "I'm placid some of the time but not all the time."

"You're placid, so you can't possibly be a passionate pianist. My best piano students have fiery personalities. One of them even throws a pencil at me when she gets frustrated." He gave me a sly grin.

"You really don't know me very well, do you?" My eyes narrowed.

"Oh, yes I do. Let's face it—I'm not your bag. I'm too impulsive for you." He looked directly at my abdomen. "Hey, you're getting a little paunchy, aren't you?"

I touched my stomach. "Only a little, and what do you expect? You've been taking me to all these fancy restaurants." He usually told me I had a perfect figure, but he was on the offensive now.

"You're very attractive but not in the classical sense. You're no Marilyn Monroe, but you know that already." He gave me a condescending smile.

I glared at him. *He claims to love me so profoundly, but he criticizes my character and my looks and doubts my musicality? Is love supposed to hurt like this?*

"You've got to play for me one day—even just a few bars," he said adamantly.

"I might play for you before I go away to grad school. I've applied to several places." I spoke with a soft voice.

"What? You should go to grad school here! You won't find a better place, and you'll never find that younger man you'll looking for," Charles said with the confidence of a clairvoyant. "And if you move in with me, I'll take care of you and make sure you finish your degree."

I gave him a half smile.

"You're giving me that mysterious smile again. God, you're gorgeous. I could make love to you right here in the boat." He shot me a seductive look.

You don't truly love me, but you crave my body. I paused before I spoke. I dipped my hand in the sunray-dappled, greenish-brown water and watched a gray-blue heron land in a tall evergreen on the nearby shore. The prehistoric-looking bird squawked as it landed. I admired its graceful freedom and wanted to fly away with it. I felt that nature loved me infinitely more than Charles ever would.

"That wouldn't be a good idea." I was firm as I continued to watch the heron. I hoped I would find someone who would be so at peace with himself and who would so fully accept himself that he wouldn't compare himself with anyone else and would be optimistic and cheerful most of the time. *And even if I don't find anyone like that, maybe I'll learn to love and accept myself so much that I'll be perfectly content with my own company and will be thrilled to sit in a boat alone and watch herons land in trees.*

Chapter 12

The Music of the Spheres

I studied piano with an incredible teacher at the Cleveland Institute of Music. He had two fabulous grand pianos in his studio, placed side by side under a picture window.

After playing a few pages of Chopin's "Ballade in G minor" for him before my first lesson, he said, "You're good, but you need to learn how to play legato and to bring out the rhythm more."

"Thanks for telling me you think I'm good," I beamed.

He grinned at me and then shared one of the most profound insights I've ever heard: "We're all big kids at heart, no matter how old we get. That inner kid is just beneath the surface. We all need an encouraging pat on the back, and we all want to feel safe."

I gazed at him with wide eyes. *We're all big kids. He's right.*

He told me to buy urtext (pure text) versions of some of Haydn's pieces, saying that these were the preferred teaching tools of the Kiev school of piano teaching. Since his own piano teacher at the Institute had studied in Kiev, he felt very comfortable with this method.

I brought them to my next lesson, and then he unlocked the

biggest secret of good playing. "Rhythm is the most fundamental aspect of music," he said. "You can have rhythm without a melody, but you can't have melody without rhythm." He paused to let that sink in. "Just try singing 'Happy Birthday' without rhythm and see how far you get. And if you think about it, you'll see that rhythm is everywhere in the natural world as well."

I thought about it. "Of course," I said in a pensive tone. "Rhythm is everywhere. Our hearts beat rhythmically. There's the rhythm of day and night, the seasons, the years, and all that."

He nodded, obviously happy that I got his point and agreed with him.

"Now, look at this Haydn piece," he said as he pointed to the music I had in front of me. "You could be the most musical person in the world, but if you aren't aware of the importance of emphasizing the strong downbeats more than the weaker beats, your playing would always be missing that special quality that makes it super good. Passion and technique are not enough to really play well. You have to bring out the rhythmic importance of each note as well."

He demonstrated by playing the first few bars and then asked me to imitate him.

I tried, and I felt like a baby learning how to walk all over again.

"Ha, don't worry about it; it happens to everyone when they first realize what they should have been doing all along." He smiled at me reassuringly.

I looked at my fingers and sighed. "This is hard. And I like to play too fast anyway."

He laughed sympathetically. "Dizh poor girrl hazh so many prroblemz," he said with a mock Ukrainian-German-Jewish accent, his blue eyes shining under his curly brown hair.

Then I also laughed and had to suppress my giggling while attempting to play again.

After we worked on the Haydn pieces for a few weeks, he told me he was thrilled with my progress. "You have no idea how happy this makes me," he said with ebullient enthusiasm. "You've come such a long way in just a few weeks, it's almost unbelievable." He gave me a sunny grin.

I sat up straight. "Really? I'm so glad you think so."

"Oh, I know so." And then he continued with two life-changing, inspiring comments I'll never forget. "If you had been properly trained since early childhood, you would have been able to do absolutely anything as a pianist."

I felt as if I had sprouted wings and was flying up toward a double rainbow.

And when it was time for me to play for him, he said, "Now remember, anything is possible. There are no limits." He smiled at me as if he were my very best friend.

I often think of his words, "Anything is possible," when I compose music. Those words unleashed the courage I needed to be creative and to realize my musical dreams. What a blessing it is to meet those angels in life—those people who infuse you with love, light, and life. Even one of these angels can give you the armor to protect yourself against a horde of negative people who are not empathic toward you. We all have the potential to be someone's angel. One genuine smile, one kind word, or one warm hug can lift another person out of depression or even give him or her the courage to start a new life.

Astronomers, using high-tech instruments, have recently shown that the music of the spheres was not just an ancient cosmic dream. When I visited the American Museum of Natural History in New York a few years ago, I saw a fascinating display about the sun. It has internal vibrations that are way beyond our hearing range, but if these vibrations were converted so we could actually hear them, we would hear octaves. Music could be an expression of the life force.

Maybe there is a cosmic "Ode to Joy" playing in the heavens right now, urging us to love and accept ourselves and everyone else and to create a better life on earth.

Chapter 13

Pierre and the Older Woman

I was elated to be sitting beside Pierre in the backseat of a stretch limo that was taking us to a swanky downtown hotel for an evening of dinner and dancing. The windows were half open, letting in the mild mid-November air. What a fascinating guy. He was a good med student, but he had so many other interests we'd never run out of things to talk about. I wondered, *How could anyone be more multifaceted than he is? And he's got those intelligent, laughing eyes and a smile to match. He'll make an ideal family physician.*

"You've got such a great laugh," Pierre said. "It's so infectious that it makes me happy."

"Good! Many people tell me the same thing. I was born this way. Even when I was only two years old, Mom says total strangers got a real kick out of me in stores and would tell her: 'Look at that funny, cross-eyed kid.'"

"I wish I could be like that more often," Pierre said in a serious tone.

"Oh, come on! You were the life of the Halloween party, all

dressed up as a French clown and acting so crazy. You made everyone laugh, including my parents," I said in a lighthearted voice.

"I see a psychiatrist every few weeks because I'm always looking for the same woman—a woman who's just like my mother. My father is a military officer who was away a lot when I was a kid, so I got too attached to my mom, and when he was home, he was way too strict and critical."

I was stunned. I was amazed that he was honest enough to bare his soul like this on a first date, but the fact that he had to see a psychiatrist at such a young age was not an auspicious sign. He appeared to be such a fantastic guy, and I enjoyed his company immensely, but I feared he would be too unpredictable for me. I had endured extreme stress in my life, but I didn't need a psychiatrist to help me cope with it. (Later on in my life, I realized that getting psychiatric help is an admirable act of self-preservation.)

I wondered whether there had been any subtle signs of Pierre's emotional troubles at the Halloween party where we first met. He looked so funny, wearing a little green felt bowler hat and bright green tights. His face was hidden under a thick coat of white paint decorated with black spades and clubs and red diamonds. His white and black pirate shirt added an adventurous Jean Lafitte-like flair to his comical appearance.

People made a wide circle around him to watch him make sweeping windmill-like gestures with his arms, walk up imaginary stairs, and lean on nonexistent railings. His performance was riveting.

When he took a break, I asked him where he learned to mime so well.

"I took a mime course out west last summer," he said. "I rode my bike there and back and had a great time." He was very upbeat.

"You rode your bike all that way?" I asked, wide-eyed.

"Yeah, he did," said another medical student who was dressed as a hobo, complete with a front tooth painted black to make it look like it was missing, a tattered flannel plaid shirt, faded jeans, and a six-pack of beer attached to the frayed rope around his waist. "I've come prepared!" he said, ripping off a can of beer from the plastic ring holder and held it high.

Pierre smirked at the hobo and said, "You're a perfect ten. You're a four with a six-pack."

"I'm a helluva lot more than that, you clown." The hobo was not to be dismissed so casually. "And you wait until I become a surgeon and operate on you."

Pierre ignored him and touched my turquoise earrings. "Those are really pretty. Do you want to dance?" His eyes looked playful and hopeful even through the heavy makeup.

"Sure," I said as Pierre led me to the center of the room. Someone put on the dance music, and we were joined by a sexy lady vampire, a tomato, a pumpkin, Kermit, the king of hearts, and many others. I loved Pierre's sizzling energy and enjoyed dancing with him and watching the others have such a riotously good time all around me. I nearly doubled over laughing when the song Monster Mash started.

"Do you want to go out some time?" Pierre asked me when the dance ended. He sounded really hopeful.

"I'd love to," I said with controlled enthusiasm. I didn't want Pierre to know how ecstatic I really was that he had asked me out. I wouldn't have recognized him without his makeup, but I was really excited about going out with him.

The limo stopped in front of the hotel, hurling me back into the present. Pierre led me into the huge convention room that was reserved for the dinner and dance.

"I did my first year of college in Europe," Pierre told me as we approached a table loaded with appetizers. "And I want to see as much of the world as possible. Actually, I think it would be great to sail around the world. With the right people to sail with, it would be a lot of fun." He looked very determined.

"I love to travel too," I said. "What an exhilarating adventure it would be to sail around the world." I could almost feel the sea wind in my hair and wondered what it would be like to travel with him.

We danced for hours after dinner, and when the event was over, the limo took us back to my house.

Pierre walked with me along the oak-lined driveway. The only light came from a distant flickering street lamp. When we arrived at the door, Pierre said, "I had a really, really good time!"

I nodded. "I did too."

"We'll have to do this again sometime," he said as he squeezed my hand.

"Sure," I said. I liked his warm, strong grip. His hands looked like a kind doctor's hands, even in the dark.

Pierre walked back down the driveway, and the limo drove him away. I was overwhelmed with competing feelings of joy, hope, and despair. I had just been on the most enjoyable date of my life, but the sickening image of Pierre going to a psychiatrist almost choked me as I entered the house.

In mid-December, Pierre invited me to an evening Christmas party held at the ageing and neglected old mansion he and several other students were renting. Many boisterous people were already there when I arrived. It was great to hear so much carefree laughter, and I stopped to admire the wreath hanging on the door knocker. It was interwoven with Spanish moss and oyster shells.

"Merry Christmas! Come on in." Pierre was jovial as he led me through the living room crowd and into the kitchen. "I've made my special, extra-hot jambalaya. It's almost ready." The aroma of spicy sausage, chicken, prawns, and rice wafted up from the hot stove.

"You cook too?" I was very impressed.

Pierre nodded and gave a Gallic shrug.

"What would you like to drink?" A man who looked like the Halloween hobo was the bartender, standing next to a table full of bottles.

"I remember you," I said. "You were the one with the six pack." I grinned.

"That's right, but I don't look so ridiculous tonight. Good to see you."

"I'll have a bit of red wine, please."

The hobo poured some wine into a little plastic glass and gave it to me.

Pierre had gone back into the big living room to mingle with the crowd.

The hobo beckoned to me, so I moved closer to him. "That Pierre is a really mixed-up guy. He falls madly in love with a girl—madly, madly in love." He paused dramatically. "And then he gets sick of them."

"Is that right?" I whispered. I didn't know whether to believe him or not, but I began to understand why Pierre had to see a psychiatrist.

Pierre was organizing everyone in the living room, preparing them to sing carols.

The hobo rolled his eyes and chuckled. "We have to go in there and sing. He won't leave us alone until we go in there and sing."

I joined the others in the living room. They sang some carols, and I enjoyed watching Pierre direct everyone with theatrical flair, as if he were on stage.

When he had enough directing, he went back in the kitchen and brought out the jambalaya.

I tasted it. "Wow, that's the hottest thing I've ever had." I breathed out hard and fanned my mouth with my hand. Then I sipped some wine to dilute the hellish Tabasco sauce.

"Hey, how many bottles of that red stuff did you put in there?" someone asked.

Pierre shrugged and put on some dance music. "Hey, everybody, let's dance."

Several couples started dancing, and then Pierre asked me to dance with him.

After half an hour, Pierre and I were the only ones dancing. And after another fifteen minutes, Pierre was flat on the floor, pretending to have fainted, and I was still standing.

"That's the first time we've ever seen anyone outlast Pierre," some people shouted.

"Way to go," someone said to me. "Not bad for an older woman. You're a lot older than Pierre, aren't you?"

"Yes, I'm four years older," I said as I looked down at Pierre. I smiled, but I didn't appreciate being called an older woman. I was only twenty-eight, and Pierre was twenty-four. I suppose I would have been admired even more if I had been nineteen. A woman can never be young enough.

I helped Pierre up, and everyone cheered.

When it was time for me to leave, Pierre gave me some beautiful framed photographs of sunsets. "These are for you. I took them when I went camping a few weeks ago."

"These look professional," I said. "What lovely colors. Thanks."

Pierre gave me a long, warm hug. "See you soon," he said. His hug felt so good and so right, even after what the hobo told me in the kitchen and even though I had been called an older woman.

"Yes, and thanks for the great party," I said as I stepped out the door.

"So when are you going to move in?" Pierre asked me casually when everyone else was out of earshot.

I just smiled at him, knowing he had had too much to drink.

I woke up in the middle of the night with a thumping heart. "Oh, how dreadful," I whispered. I had a lurid dream of a cavalier

Pierre, his face painted white, dressed as a clown, and dancing with five adoring young women. I was not psychic, but my dreams were sometimes prophetic.

Pierre asked me to spend a day in the country with him, so on one warm spring morning, we drove on curvy country roads through a mixed forest and arrived at a big lake surrounded by thick bright green pines. There was a small, lonely concession stand on the beach.

We waded in the shallow water and swam slowly toward a deeper area. After treading water for a little while, Pierre shot off like a flying fish, performing the butterfly stroke with the agility and fearsome strength of an Olympic athlete, slapping the water and creating lots of foamy waves. I didn't even try to keep up with him, and he was far away in seconds. I was amazed at his strength and agility.

When Pierre finally swam back to me, he told me he was hungry.

"I'm hungry too. Let's go to the stand," I said. "The way you swam, I'm not surprised you're hungry."

We ordered chili dogs and coffee and sat down on a picnic table under the pines. I could hear a train in the distance. "You remember those train tracks beside my house?" Pierre asked me. "Sometimes when I get bummed out and I hear the passing trains, I imagine jumping on board, going far away, and leaving everything behind. Then I feel better. I want to be a professional hobo."

"Have you told your father about that? What would he think?" I was taken aback.

"He says I should be a military doctor with a straight and narrow, regimented life."

"I can't see you in a regimented life of any kind," I said.

"Thanks. That's why I'm into civilian family practice. I believe in preventive medicine and living a really healthy life to avoid getting sick in the first place."

"And if everyone would be even half as physically active as you are, they probably would avoid getting sick in the first place. I can't believe how well you swam out there. I thought I was a good swimmer, but you're too much." My eyes widened.

Pierre chewed his food with a contagiously nervous energy. "I'm learning how to walk on a tightrope too. There's one strung up between the trees back at the house, and I practice on it. It's at least eight feet up."

"Maybe you can show it to me when we get back to your place," I said. I finished my coffee and the chili dog.

The other students and some of their friends were sitting in the backyard when Pierre and I got back to the house. Everyone whistled and clapped when Pierre quickly scrambled from one end of the tightrope to the other without a balancing aid of any kind. He behaved as if he were invincible.

Pierre jumped down and smiled at me.

"That was terrific, but I've got to go now," I said.

Pierre gave me a light kiss on the cheek. "That was a fun day. See you soon."

We went out for a gourmet dinner and a sci-fi adventure movie a couple of weeks later and had a wonderful time. He was charismatic and full of life.

That night I had a dream about him. He was white-faced again, but he was dancing alone.

I went to a dinner party at a friend's apartment a few weeks later and met a motherly, middle-aged librarian who apparently knew Pierre quite well.

"Pierre comes into the library quite often to confide in me," I overheard the lady say to the hostess in the living room while we were enjoying predinner cocktails.

I got a little queasy.

"He says he's lonely because he doesn't have a girlfriend."

I felt as if I had just swallowed a hand grenade, but I didn't say a word.

"I've seen Pierre walking down the street with some lovely young women, so I don't understand why he says he's so lonely," the lady said.

I remembered the dreams. I was just an observer in those dreams, and that's all I was in his life. I didn't mean anything to him. I felt like kicking myself for being attracted to him and for craving his company. I felt that the clown had turned me into a total fool.

Pierre called me a couple of months later and asked if he could listen to me practice piano at a nearby college.

"Well ... sure. If you really want to ..." I was amazed at his eagerness.

"I'm really looking forward to it!"

"Oh, good. See you at seven then." I managed to sound calm, but I was very pleased to hear from him. The liveliness in his voice always excited me and made me think of adventures in faraway lands. After all, he wanted to sail around the world.

Pierre sat quietly while I played some of my piano compositions and then clapped loudly at the end. "You've got something unique there," he said fervently while giving me an admiring look. "And I think the world of you and your parents."

I was slack-jawed, but I managed a weak smile.

"I'm going back east to take a short course at another university, and I want to see you when I get back," he said as he held my arms with possessive affection. "Maybe we can go hiking in the woods and see your parents' cabin on the lake."

I looked deep into his eyes, and he seemed to be very sincere—so sincere, in fact, that it made me question everything I had heard about him. He was gripping my arms with such strength that I felt he couldn't possibly be dangerously confused. It was the grip of a man who knew what he wanted. Or did he?

When I heard that Pierre was back, I called him and asked if he still wanted to go for a hike and see the cabin.

"Sure, I'd love to. I've always wanted to see that place," he said cheerfully.

"Oh, good. How about this weekend?" I always loved going there.

"That will work. Great! By the way, can I bring my girlfriend along?"

Even though I felt that Zeus had just zapped me with a custom lightning bolt designed to crush my spirit, I managed to speak with a steady voice and tell him it was okay for him to bring her. I didn't want to appear to be jealous. I never wanted to give that impression to anyone.

I drove to the cabin on Saturday morning, and Pierre and his girlfriend arrived just before noon. She was a lovely young woman, and she gave me a shy smile. When Pierre went back to the car and was out of earshot, she said, "Pierre is amazing. He's so good at everything, and I feel so dumb beside him. I'm just fresh out of high school, and he'll be a doctor soon."

"Yes, he is amazing," I said.

"I've heard wonderful things about you," she said. "He really admires you."

"What? Really?" I must have looked totally perplexed.

Pierre came back from the car, took his girlfriend's hand, and led her to the water's edge.

"You two can explore while I make lunch," I called out to them.

"Okay," Pierre said as they stripped down to their bathing suits, jumped in the lake, and swam around the boathouse.

I put some steaks on the gas grill beside the cabin and went inside to make a salad.

Pierre and his friend emerged from the lake just in time for lunch on the porch.

"This is really good. Thank you," she said.

"Yes, thank you," Pierre said.

After lunch, the three of us went for a long walk in the woods close to the lake. We saw a blue heron spread its enormous wings and take off from a gray log on the beach, and a few minutes later we saw a red fox leap across our path and disappear into the woods. When we reached a narrow paved road, a big blond buck with huge antlers charged out of the forest, bounced on the road with a clickety-clack sound, and ploughed its way through the forest on the other side.

"Those animals sure seem to know what they're after, don't they? They all move with this purposeful energy," I said.

"Yes, they do," Pierre's friend said.

"Some of us are a lot more mixed up than they are, including me," Pierre said softly.

We walked back to the cabin.

"Thanks so much for everything," Pierre's friend said in a subdued tone.

"This place is even more beautiful than I imagined it to be," Pierre said. "Thanks."

Pierre and his friend sped off in their car, and then I checked the cabin, locked up, and walked toward my car. As I looked back at the lake, I thought, *How I love coming here. Nature is a healer and helps me keep things in perspective. And it doesn't judge me for being an older woman.*

That night, I dreamt of a fearless white-faced Pierre walking on a tightrope.

A few months later, when Pierre was doing his internship, I received a beautiful handwritten letter from him saying that he missed me and my parents. I read it over and over, hoping his words were sincere. Even though the girlfriend I met at the lake was just a teenager and I was an older woman, I was still hoping he was sincere.

A few weeks after that, I was looking at a bulletin board in the entrance hall of the college music building where I sometimes practiced when I felt a tap on my shoulder. I turned to face a pleasant-looking young man.

"Remember me? I met you at that funny Halloween party a while back."

I studied his face for a few seconds and then smiled. "Oh, yes … yes. I do remember you! You were dressed as the king of hearts. You were in Pierre's class, and you came to his parties at the mansion." I paused. "By the way, how is Pierre?"

"Oh, you haven't heard?" The young man's voice softened.

"No." I became a little lightheaded.

"He was skiing with a bunch of friends when an avalanche started coming down the mountain. His friends managed to get out of the way, but he seemed to think he could ski faster than the avalanche. They screamed at him and told him to get out of the way, but he didn't make it."

"Oh my God!"

"They've never found his body."

Pierre might have been confused, but he was unforgettable. And he didn't deserve to die young.

Going to a psychiatrist and being so honest about it showed an admirable desire for self-acceptance and self-preservation.

Now that I have learned to fully love and accept myself, I no longer care when anyone calls me an older woman. I'm just sorry that we live in a global society that glorifies youth and often ignores the beautiful gifts older people can offer.

Chapter 14

Ralph

"I'm thinking of suspending Ralph for a week," my principal told me in a gloomy tone of voice as he leaned back in his chair. "He's one of those boys who doesn't respond to any of the positive reinforcements we throw at him. None of the middle schools can handle him, so the head office, in its infinite wisdom, sends him to us."

The principal rolled his eyes and sighed so hard that the pencil on his desk rolled toward the edge and fell off. "Aaargh!" He bent down, picked it up, and slammed it back down on the desk. "Sorry," he said, grinning. "I'm not usually this frustrated, but Ralphy-Boy is something else." He gave me an inquiring look. "How does he behave when he comes to your music class?"

"Amazingly enough, he loves to sing. He forgets about bullying the other kids when it's time to sing a familiar song or learn a new one." I spoke in a positive tone and then paused to think. "Hmmm." I thought some more. "You know, tomorrow afternoon I'm taking a few of the choir kids over to a nursing home that's just a few blocks away. The staff called and said the residents are really excited and can't wait to hear us sing Christmas carols. Maybe I should take Ralph along and see how he does."

"Great idea! I hope he does okay, because I would hate to suspend him so close to Christmas. He might get into some really serious trouble because there's no one at home to keep him in line except his poor old great-grandma."

"Oh! The parents are working, are they?" I looked hopeful.

"Hell no. His father's in jail for selling drugs, and his mom's a hooker. I guess she works, ha, ha."

"No wonder all I get is a thin little voice whenever I call his house …"

"Good luck tomorrow," he said, laughing.

"Thanks," I replied with a chuckle. "I'll make him carry the keyboard over there, so he'll have an important job to do and won't be able to punch anybody."

"Let me know how it goes," he said. "Do you need a police escort?"

I shook with laughter as I got up and left his office.

* * * * *

"Ralph, will you please carry the keyboard over to the nursing home? I know you're really strong." I nodded encouragingly at him and gave him a maternal smile the next afternoon as the selected choir singers and I got ready to leave the music room. We had just finished a good vocal warm-up and were looking forward to the short walk over there.

"Oh, yeah." Ralph flexed his muscles like a pro boxer. "I'm strong." He grabbed the keyboard and held it firmly.

"Thanks!" I grinned at him, and he gave me a grateful half smile.

Ralph behaved perfectly all the way to the home, even whistling and singing some of the carols. And he didn't drop the keyboard.

Soon after we arrived, the staff directed us to the activity room close to the front door, and we got set up. Ralph gingerly placed the keyboard on a table, plugged it in, and joined the other singers around the instrument. I placed the piano music on the table stand and got ready to play "Jingle Bell Rock."

There were about twenty residents there, some sitting on couches, some in wooden chairs, and some in wheelchairs. Most were in pajamas and housecoats, and they were all hushed with anticipation. Even though many were gazing at us with clouded eyes, their enthusiasm shone through.

"Hit it, girlie," a bent lady in curlers said in a cracked voice.

I gave a broad smile, played the short intro, and sang along with the kids, who came in on cue.

Ralph stood next to me and sang his young tuneful heart out, his voice projecting over all the others and his body swaying to the catchy rhythm. It was as if someone had plugged him in and he had finally discovered what it meant to be vivaciously, ecstatically alive.

Even though the residents were struggling with the ravaging cruelty of old age, they forgot about their aches and pains and clapped joyfully. Some had tears streaming down their faces, and others had beatific smiles that made them look twenty years younger.

Ralph stood up straight, beamed, and whispered to me, "They love us, they love us. When do we start the next song?"

"Right away," I murmured. "You're terrific, Ralph."

We sang for about half an hour, and the residents and the staff were thrilled the whole time. Ralph sang every song with the same fantastic energy, and everyone looked forward to our return.

I didn't have to ask Ralph to carry the keyboard back to the school; he grabbed it and sang all the way back. The other kids sang too, and some people waved at us from their cars as they passed us. Others leaned out of windows and cheered, "Merry Christmas!"

The principal didn't suspend Ralph, and he behaved passably for the rest of the school year.

On the last day of school, Ralph told me he had joined the youth choir at his great-grandma's church and was also singing in a rock band. He said he wanted to make a living as a car mechanic but that he would keep singing for the rest of his life. The gratitude of the old folks at Christmas made him realize that it was much more fun to rock on than to beat people up. He didn't have to do that anymore to prove himself; all he had to do was sing as loud as he could and be admired and appreciated for it.

Chapter 15

Frank

"Hey, look at Frank!" One of my students pointed at the classroom windows, so I looked up from my desk and saw Frank walking outside with his distinctive macho swagger. *Why isn't he in my class?* I wondered.

I rushed over to the classroom door, but Frank had already reached the next classroom by the time I opened the door. "Frank?" I called.

"Huh?" He looked back at me but kept on walking. *What's he up to now?*

I spotted Frank in the school yard during afternoon recess and approached him. "Why were you just walking around instead of coming to math and science class today? You missed an important lesson." I frowned at him anxiously.

"Sorry, ma'am, but sometimes I just can't sit still. I have to get up and walk around." He looked down at the cracked blacktop, his dark, curly hair full of sunlight.

"Oh, you're so restless you have to go on a walkabout," I said.

"You mean like those Australian aborigines or something?" he asked with a serious voice.

"Good for you for knowing about aborigines, Frank. And yes, that's what I mean by walkabout. Some people just have to get away from any kind of routine, but you can't escape it forever." I put my hand on his shoulder with a gentle touch.

"I'll come to class tomorrow," he said in a convincing tone.

"Good! See you tomorrow." I gave him an approving smile.

Frank was in my introductory algebra class the next morning. I told the students that the famous Einstein had trouble with algebra until an uncle told him he should think of it as "chasing Mr. X."

"I'm going to call myself Mr. X from now on," Frank blurted out. He was sitting at a round table with another boy and four giggling, love-struck girls.

Even though he hadn't raised his hand to ask permission to speak, I didn't scold him because I was happy he showed such a strong interest in algebra.

"Mr. X, that sounds cool," one boy whispered.

"Mr. X, yeah, yeah," a soft whisper snaked around the room from student to student.

Frank is a born leader in spite of his need for the occasional walkabout.

Close to the end of class, I let the students work on a few algebra problems and told them to raise a hand if they finished before the bell so I could check their work. Frank's hand shot up quickly. I walked over to him, and saw that he had solved everything correctly. "Terrific," I said. "You sure know how to chase Mr. X, and that's not easy." I smiled down at him.

"Thanks, ma'am," Frank said. No other hands went up before the bell, and the instant it rang, they were ready to leap out to the next class.

During junior high science class a week later, we discussed our ancestors.

"According to many scientists, human beings originated in Africa and spread out to other continents from there. No matter how different we may look on the surface, we all have similar DNA structures," I said. I showed the class some drawings of the DNA double helix and then asked if anyone wanted to share information about their ancestry.

"I'm Hispanic and white," said one lovely girl with wavy hair.

"I'm African American and Native American," said a dark-skinned boy.

"I'm from Vietnam," said a boy with hooded eyes and thin black hair.

"What are you, Frank?" A boy sitting at Frank's table was very curious, and so was everyone else. They all turned to look at him.

"I'm a mix," Frank said. "A real mix."

"What kind of mix?" another boy asked. It was hard to tell what Frank really was.

"I've got everything in me—some black, some white, some Asian, and some Latino."

"Awesome," squealed the girl who was sitting across from him.

"I'm the human of the future," said Frank with an authoritative voice. "I've read that in a few decades, we'll all be as mixed as I am. There aren't that many whites even now, and they'll disappear one day. Everyone will eventually look pretty much the same."

"No way," said one boy.

"Oh, yeah? The scientists say so, and we wouldn't have anything without them. Not even phones." He was very sure of himself and gave a smug smile.

I smiled to myself. Frank looked like a James Dean–type rebel with his worn leather jacket, but he was a real thinker with great potential.

After the discussion, I asked the students to look through the microscopes at their tables and draw the human blood cells that were on the prepared slides.

"Hey, I just thought of another thing," Frank said after he raised his hand. "We all have red blood, no matter what color our skin is." He looked very pleased with himself.

Everyone sat up straight, as if a huge light bulb had suddenly appeared over the entire class.

I walked around the room to see the drawings and was pleased to see all the students diligently trying to draw exactly what they saw. Frank's drawing was full of accurate details.

When class was over, I asked Frank to stay behind.

"Ma'am?" he asked, looking a little worried.

"Nothing to worry about, Frank, calm down." When the rest of the students were gone, I looked into his eyes. "Frank, you have a good scientific mind. I'm amazed at how smart you are. You know, if you keep applying yourself and never give up on school, you'll be able to get a really good job and go far in life. I really mean that." I spoke with a firm, encouraging tone.

Frank nodded and turned his head away. "Can I go now?"

"Okay." I wasn't sure if I had managed to influence him or not, but it felt good to try.

A week later, I spotted Frank and his best buddy pretending to fight on the playground during Friday afternoon recess. "Kiss mah butt," they sneered at each other as other students cheered them on.

They stopped play-fighting when they saw me walking toward them. "So what plans do you two have for this long weekend?" I smiled at them when I stood next to them.

"Blowing up houses in Pasadena," they said without hesitation.

"You must be joking," I said.

"No, ma'am, we ain't joking." They both looked determined.

Frank stood tall and said, "I'm a tough guy. I ain't no nerd." He punched the air.

His buddy, kicking a pebble, said, "I'm tough too."

"I'm tougher," said Frank as he gave the air a one-two punch.

His buddy was quiet.

After the long weekend, Frank came to my class wearing a blue bandanna.

The next day, all the kids showed up wearing something blue. Some wore blue shoes, some wore blue belts, and some girls carried blue purses. One boy wore a single blue glove.

The principal sent me a note asking me to see her after school. "I'm very worried about Frank," she said to me in her office.

"I'm worried about him too," I said. "Is it because of the blue colors he's wearing?"

"That's right. I can't prove it, but I think he's joined a gang in LA. He's not just a wannabe anymore."

"That's horrible. I've talked to him and told him what a great future he has if he finishes school, but he seems to prefer playing the macho man."

"Of course. These boys are so insecure to begin with, and joining a gang feeds their ego and makes them feel like they're somebody. We've got to watch him closely."

"I'll talk to him again," I said.

"I've scheduled a conference with his mother," the principal said.

* * * * *

Frank continued to shine in my math and science classes and got very good grades at the end of the school year. I wished him luck, knowing he would go to another school in the fall.

A couple of years later, I was casually perusing the local paper when I thought I recognized Frank's full name. I read it and reread it and reread it again. "Our dear, beloved Frank was shot on the street close to our house on Sunday afternoon. The family would like to thank the paramedics and emergency room doctors for trying so hard to save his life. There will be a memorial service for close friends and family at the house."

I put my head in my hands and let out a deep, tortured groan. *Poor, poor Frank. Why did you have to leave us so soon? You were barely fifteen years old. Why, oh, why did you have to be seduced by those gangs? You didn't need a blue bandanna and a gun to prove yourself—not with your superbright mind. I cared about you and I miss you terribly, Mr. X.*

Chapter 16

Charmaine

"You might as well just take her home," the young internist said in a matter-of-fact tone of voice. "She'll die in a couple of days at the most. There's nothing more we can do."

I let out a long, tortured sigh. Mom's abdomen was frightfully distended to at least five times its normal size, as if she were pregnant with quintuplets, and the attached drain bag was bulging with a dark reddish-brown liquid that made me wonder if her liver was liquefying and disintegrating. I was glad she was asleep in her hospital bed, oblivious to the doctor's fatalistic pronouncements.

"But … but … can't you give her a liver transplant? Some people get those, don't they?" I was frantic. Mom was more like a vulnerable sister than a mother to me, and I felt very protective toward her.

"No way. Hardly anyone qualifies for a liver transplant." He shook his head.

I gave another tortured sigh. "How am I going to handle her all by myself? My father is in a nursing home because he had a massive stroke, and now he has congestive heart failure on top of that. I'm an only child, and I don't have any relatives who can help out." I spoke in a firm, urgent tone, hoping he would understand my impossible situation.

"You could speak to the social worker about getting some nursing help, although it's going to be hard on such short notice." He seemed nonchalant as he gave me a casual glance.

I rolled my eyes and groaned.

"I have to finish my rounds now." He shook my hand. "Good luck."

Thanks a million, I thought as he left the room. The midafternoon sun was streaming in from the third-floor window, but it didn't warm anything.

"Mom? Mom?" I whispered as I touched her blanket. She was still asleep, her enormous abdomen rising and falling with each weak breath. When the caring emergency room doctor examined her a few days before she was admitted, he had told me that her ascites was caused by liver cirrhosis and that when alcoholics drink heavily for years, they destroy their livers. He thought Mom's condition was hopeless. However, even though two doctors had already given up on her, I couldn't accept that her time had come. *My dear Mom.* She fled from Stalin's holocaust in 1944 and sat alone on her brown metal suitcase at the railway station trying to escape the firebombing of Dresden. Second generation children of holocaust survivors often echo their parents' pain. My mother's pain was my pain.

I walked down the hall to the nurse's station and asked them if I could speak to a social worker.

"She should be back from her break any second now," a nurse said as she continued to fill out some forms behind the counter.

The young social worker was very helpful, giving me the name and phone number of a private nursing company and arranging for a transfer ambulance to take Mom home.

I rushed out to the crowded hospital parking lot and then drove home to wait for the ambulance and to call for a private nurse. They answered right away and said they would send someone to the house the next day. I was grateful for that, but I didn't know how I would cope until then.

The ambulance crew brought Mom back on a stretcher, and I directed them to her bedroom. Their job was relatively easy because we had a comfortable ranch home. They worked quickly, and I thanked them profusely. I didn't want them to leave, but they had to rush back to the hospital.

"Mom, are you okay?" I asked as I stood beside her and looked into her big blue-gray eyes. Her matted blonde hair looked as if it was begging to be washed. The ominous drain with the iodine-dark liquid hung beside the bed. She was usually fearless, but her eyes betrayed the terror in her heart as she tried to shift in her bed. All she could manage was a slight wiggle, so she cried and sniffed like a little girl who had fallen off her bike and scraped her knees. "I feel horrible," she said as she fumbled with the abdominal drain, trying to disconnect it.

"No! You can't do that," I said as I secured the drain. "You need that drain for now." *How am I going to survive until the nurse comes? I was totally exhausted even before she went to the hospital.*

I may have had four hours of poor sleep that night, and in the morning I dragged myself over to Mom's room. She was staring at the ceiling and holding her abdomen. *She's still alive. Now where's the nurse? My kingdom for a nurse.*

"I'm thirsty," Mom whispered. "I need water."

"I'll bring you a glass," I said.

No matter how hard Mom tried to sit up, she couldn't do it. Her abdomen was so heavy it anchored her in place. "Mmph, mmph," she sighed and whimpered.

I put the glass on her lips, hoping she could at least have a sip of water, but she turned her head away.

Then the doorbell rang. I leaped out of the bedroom and opened the front door.

"Good morning. You called for a nurse? I'm Charmaine."

"Yes! Oh, yes! I called! I need help with my mom! Come in. Please come in."

I led Charmaine into the kitchen and quickly told her what the internist and the emergency room doctor had said about Mom and that Dad was terminally ill and in a nursing home. I kept my voice soft so Mom would not hear.

"You're coping with both parents, as ill as they are, with no one to talk to?" She drew a sharp breath, and her intense blue eyes widened. Her light blonde hair was pulled back and piled up on top of her head. She was tall, slender, and as graceful as a ballerina and projected profound concern.

"The nursing home staff does a great job with Dad, and I always enjoy talking to them when I visit, but I've been too busy caregiving to make friends here. It's tough to do this alone."

"Shall we see your mother now?" Charmaine spoke softly.

I nodded and led her to Mom's room.

"Who are you? What's going on?" Mom looked at Charmaine and me with suspicion.

"Mom, this is Charmaine. She's a nurse, and she's here to help us out for a while."

"Why?" Mom still looked suspicious.

I leaned over and stroked her matted hair. "Because you're very ill, and we want to help you get better. I can't do everything by myself anymore."

"Hello, Madame. I'm here to help." Charmaine smiled at Mom and gently pulled the covers away from her abdomen. There were several nasty-looking, oozing sores. "I'll clean up your abdomen, if that's okay," Charmaine said, sounding very sweet and soothing.

"I'll get a washcloth and bowl." I wasted no time getting them.

Charmaine cleaned up the sores and emptied the drain bag. She seemed to enjoy her work, in spite of the pungent odors that wafted up from the bed.

"You have very kind hands," Mom told her as she looked into her eyes.

I was relieved that Mom didn't seem to be so suspicious anymore. Mom was loved by most, but she sometimes behaved like a bull in a china shop. One male admirer called her a "kick in the pants."

When Mom was all cleaned up and ready for a rest, Charmaine looked at me and tilted her head in the direction of the kitchen.

We sat across from each other at the kitchen dinette table. "She's *not* dying." She was adamant.

"She's not?" I was incredulous but hopeful.

"Absolutely not. I feel a strong life force in her body. That Dr. Death is wrong!" Charmaine looked like a dancer but spoke with the authority of a biblical prophet and the omnipotent energy of an archangel. She was supremely feminine and supremely masculine at the same time. She was fascinating and mesmerizing and exactly what I needed.

"What about the emergency room doctor?" I asked.

"Wrong too! They're *both* wrong." She was defiant. "By the way, why does your mother drink so much?" Now she spoke with gentle concern.

"She's been very depressed and anxious for years, and she's self-medicating. Many doctors, here and in the States, have urged her to stop and to see a psychiatrist. She refuses, saying she wants to die and that this is the way she wants to go. Sometimes when I get really firm with her and try to stop her, she threatens to curse me. Dad has tried to stop her for years too, but she pays no attention to him. She'll just walk away from him before he finishes talking."

"Do you think she might be allergic to alcohol? Some people are."

"I don't know about that. I do know that she drinks huge amounts every day and refuses to get help of any kind. When I told her I joined an Al-Anon group and had to see a counselor because of her drinking, she laughed and sneered, 'Good for you.' I don't know whether to laugh or cry. Actually, I do both."

"What happened to her? Why is she so determined to harm herself?" Charmaine leaned forward and rested her chin on her hands.

I told Charmaine that Mom felt unloved, even as a child, because she was never praised as much as her older brother and sister were. Her first husband cheated her and disappeared during the war in the old country. She was born in Estonia, had to flee from the Soviets in 1944 to avoid being used as a sex slave, and was a refugee for years all by herself. Then she came to Canada without a penny, found a good job working as a nurse's aide and then as a lab technician, and met my Dad while she was working for Dr. Selye. Dad's mother never accepted Mom, however, saying she was just a poor refugee with no money and that she was "just a nurse." My father's family didn't understand why she hadn't finished her pharmacy degree in Munich. Most of the refugee students at the UNRRA university were sure Stalin would take over the whole of Germany, so she immigrated and had to work right away to survive. She was amazingly courageous in spite of her harsh fate.

Charmaine seemed to empathize completely. "Bless her heart, the poor soul." Her voice was velvety, and she shook her head slowly. "People are so quick to judge and dismiss each other. They should have praised her for doing so well on her own. We waste so much energy with our negativity, don't we?" Charmaine curled her lip in disgust.

"I know. Mom got pregnant right after she married Dad, and then she lost her health and was too busy to go back to university. She had her hands more than full with Dad and me. She didn't want to have a baby so soon, and neither did Dad. She felt trapped and had nowhere to go. She also believes that my dad doesn't love her. I understand why she drinks. It's a tragedy for our little threesome of a family, but I do understand it. It drives me crazy, though, and it's so, so sad. I get choked up when I look at her hooked up to that awful drain."

"How long has she been drinking like this?" Charmaine's eyes narrowed.

"She was okay when I was growing up. She was a good mother. The really heavy drinking started when I was in my midthirties and she was in her midsixties." I sighed.

"You should give her a B-vitamin complex. That will help her to recover."

"It's so comforting to hear you talk about recovery, but I'll have to go to the nursing home to get Dad and bring him home for a visit in case her days really are numbered. He knows what the doctors said, and he's really worried. Can you stay for a while and watch her while I go and get Dad? It won't take me long." I must have looked like a dog pleading for its dinner.

"I'll be here, don't worry." She gave me a warm, all-knowing smile.

I ignored all the speed limits on the way to the nursing home.

Dad was sitting in a chair beside a big window that overlooked a pond, an orchard, distant fields, and a glacier and was wearing his favorite navy blue tracksuit and black running shoes with Velcro straps. His left arm was bent sharply at the elbow and curled toward his chest, and the left side of his face was slightly twisted. He made a weak, staccato-like crying sound, as lefties, or people who have had a stroke in the right hemisphere of the brain, often do. I was happy he could still think and talk, but I would never have believed that a scientist with a reputation as a heart disease pioneer would end up like a pitiful, helpless baby, suffering from the very same disease he studied for so long.

"Hi, Dad. That nurse, Charmaine, is looking after Mom right now. Are you ready to go home for a while?"

"Yes, let's go." His voice was raspy, but he was lucid.

I unfolded the companion chair, helped him into it, and wheeled him out to the car. I was glad to get back out into the fresh air because the nursing home had a pervasive stale odor that was reminiscent of an overheated and overstocked used furniture store.

I paid attention to the speed limits on the way back home.

I was relieved to see Charmaine's car in front of the house, and I parked as close to the front door as possible. There were a couple of steps leading up to the door because the house was on a crawl space. Dad was unsteady on his feet and tried to regain his balance by using his cane and holding on to the rails. I was right beside him, ready to break a fall.

Dad swayed from side to side as he dragged himself to Mom's room, and cried, "I don't want to lose her yet. She's the only woman I've ever truly loved, body and soul."

Mom didn't smile. She just stared at him with wide eyes.

I knew Dad loved Mom in his own way, even though he was too ambitious, too driven, and too obsessed with his work to really show it, but I never heard him say how much he really loved her. I was truly surprised.

I introduced Dad to Charmaine, who was standing next to Mom, and then the doorbell rang. I ran to open the door.

"Hello, I'm the owner of the nursing care company." The nondescript lady shook my hand and then headed toward the dining room table with a pile of paperwork. "You're in charge of everything, aren't you?"

"Yes, please have a seat," I told her. I could hear Dad and Charmaine having a congenial and animated conversation in Mom's room.

After I filled out some forms, the supervisor asked if she could meet my parents, so I led her to Mom's room. She greeted them, and then Dad, Charmaine, and I walked back to the dining room with her.

"You're going to need a nurse for the next little while, aren't you?" the supervisor asked me.

"Yes, definitely. I can't handle this alone, as you see," I said.

"I'll see who I can send for tomorrow." She sounded as if she was in a great hurry.

Dad talked a lot to both women, and I went to check on Mom.

"I can't stand all these people in the house," Mom whined.

"It won't be too long now. Just be patient," I said as I held her hand.

The supervisor left soon after that, and Dad went back to see Mom.

"I'll take Dad back to the home very soon. Can you watch Mom just until I get back?"

"Yes, I'll be here. But I'll have to leave after you get back," Charmaine said.

I took Dad back to the nursing home and was relieved to see that Charmaine was still with Mom when I returned.

"Your Mom is resting, and she's fine. I'm sorry I have to leave now, but I sure enjoyed meeting your father! And don't worry, your mom is still strong." She exuded a soothing empathy that helped to relieve my stomach-churning anxiety.

"Thank you so much for everything," I said as I accompanied her to the door.

I prayed for a rest so I could be ready for the next crisis.

The supervisor called me in the evening to tell me she had arranged for Charmaine to come back the next morning. I had a much better night because of that.

When I opened the door at 9:00 the next morning, I saw a smiling Charmaine standing with a colorful bouquet of spring flowers. "Good morning. These are for you and your mother. I hope you like them."

"Of course! Please come in!"

"One of my specialties is flower arranging. Actually, I have worked as a florist."

I led her to Mom, who gave a slight smile when she saw the flowers.

"I arranged these just for you," Charmaine told Mom.

"Thank you. Please put them on the end table," Mom murmured.

"Would you like me to wash your hair, Madame?" Charmaine asked as she smiled at her. "I think that would help you feel a little better."

Mom nodded, and Charmaine and I went to the bathroom to get the bowl, warm water, shampoo, and towels.

Charmaine helped Mom sit up in bed and then washed her hair with a lavender-scented shampoo that dispelled the oppressive smell of sickness in the room. She finished by blow-drying Mom's hair, and some of Mom's beauty reemerged. She still had the drain attached to her, but she could move her abdomen a tiny bit more than the day before.

"I have to go to the bathroom now," she said.

I fetched the bedpan from the bathroom, and Charmaine helped Mom relieve herself.

"This is definitely a sign that you're getting better," Charmaine said after she cleaned her up.

"I want to lie down now," Mom said.

Charmaine made sure she was comfortable, and then we went to the kitchen and sat at the dinette table. It was calming to look out of the big window and the sliding patio door and see thick evergreens, rhodos, blackberry bushes, and Scotch broom.

"Your mom is not dying. In fact, she's improving already,"

Charmaine said with the confidence of a well-respected senior doctor.

I gave her a wan smile. "I'm glad you still think so." I wasn't so confident.

"Now, I must tell you that I was born with a caul. Some people call it a veil. I'm Irish Canadian, and Celts believe that babies born that way are psychic. Even when I was just a little girl, I could often see future events as if there was a television screen in front of me. My parents didn't understand me, but they tolerated me and did their best to go along with my strange behavior. I'm also very sensitive to people's soul and personality vibrations, and I don't care for my supervisor's vibes that much. She talked so much to your father yesterday that I couldn't concentrate fully on the vibes I was getting from you and your father. She was a distraction, and I was glad to get away from her."

I laughed. "Even Mom thought there were too many people here yesterday."

"As I was driving home, though, the full picture emerged. I'm fifty-five now, but when I was only twenty-four years old, I was driving alone in Vancouver one day and listening to the radio. They were interviewing your father and discussing his heart disease research, saying it was very important and that it had the potential to save a lot of lives. I was overwhelmed by a very strong feeling that I would meet your father one day! I just knew I would meet him. I told my mother about him when I got home, but she dismissed my feeling as pure wishful thinking. She knew I had been right about the future so many times, but she didn't believe this prediction."

"Wow." I was slack-jawed. "You actually have met him now."

"Yes, and when you introduced us, I remembered his unusual name. I knew I had heard that name long before I met you."

"Hey! No wonder you're so sure about my mom. Now I know why." I perked up in my chair.

"When I look at your mom, I see her as healed, smartly dressed, with a proud bearing, and walking around in beautiful places with trees and water and birds and fountains." Her eyes were scintillating.

I shook my head in awe. "Fascinating. I sure hope you're right."

She paused for quite a while. "My husband and I used to own a hobby farm in Aldergrove. We both love animals, and we had horses and chickens and geese, a goat called Charlie that used to ride in the front seat of the car with me, and even some miniature horses." She was very enthusiastic as she opened her handbag and showed me a pocket-sized album of pictures. "Here's our house, and here's our indoor pool! And here are some of my miniature horses. I think your mother would enjoy looking at these pictures."

"Oh, for sure! She grew up on a hobby farm and also lived in the big city, but she preferred the countryside, and she loves animals."

We got up and walked to Mom's room. She was awake.

"I hear you love animals," Charmaine told her. "May I show you some pictures?"

"Okay," said Mom.

Mom seemed to forget her agony for a few minutes while looking at the pictures of the horses. Charmaine and I were encouraged to see her flash a broad smile.

"I've always loved animals. Even when I was a little girl in Ontario, I would play with critters like mice and lizards in the fields. My mother would have a fit when I came home with them. She would see tails sticking out of my apron pockets, and she'd scream, 'Get that creature out of here right now!' If I saw other kids being mean to animals, I'd beat them up. 'You leave that kitty alone,' I would shout. 'How would you like it if I kicked *you* in the stomach?'"

Mom and I chuckled.

"Yes, and the older I get, the more I love animals. They can give you the kind of loyal, unconditional love that humans rarely give you. And they're not proud, selfish, or judgmental. Their souls have an innocence that so many people have lost or never had in the first place. They seem to know what's really important in this world."

"They sure do, and one of these days I'd like to get a pet or two. In the meantime, Charmaine, will you be here for a while so I can go and get my dad and bring him home for another visit?" I arched an eyebrow and nodded.

"Of course I'll be here. Don't rush. You've got enough pressure on you as it is." She gave me a reassuring smile.

"I'll be back soon with Dad, Mom," I said.

She gave a slight nod and tried to shift in her bed.

I was back with Dad in less than half an hour and helped him walk to Mom's room.

Charmaine gave him a progress report about Mom as he struggled to sit down on a chair beside the bed. He held Mom's hand and didn't cry this time.

After a few minutes, he got restless, got up, walked toward the upright piano in the living room, and sat down on the bench. Charmaine and I were beside him, making sure he wouldn't fall. I lifted the lid, and he started playing "Moscow Nights" by ear with his right hand.

Charmaine sat down beside the piano, her eyes wide with delight. When he finished, she said, "Thank you so much! I love music. I used to sing light opera in my younger days. Imagine, playing so well even with one hand."

"I'm glad you enjoyed it," he said. "My wife loves to sing, and this is one of her favorite tunes."

Charmaine and Dad discussed medicine for a while, and Dad seemed to be quite impressed with Charmaine's knowledge and experience.

Then Charmaine smiled directly at me and told my dad, "You've got a wonderful daughter, sir. I've seen how hard she tries to look after you and your wife. You're both very lucky in that way."

"Yes, I know," Dad said. "I know." He looked at me and gave me a sweet half smile.

I really appreciated Charmaine's validation of my efforts because some other people had told me that I was wasting my life as a caregiver and that I should have insisted on having my own life. They said that some women love others too much and neglect themselves in the process. I knew they had a point, but there didn't seem to be any other solution. My parents were terribly vulnerable, and there was no one else to protect them.

Dad got up from the piano bench with great difficulty, walked back to Mom's room, and stayed with her while Charmaine and I talked in the living room.

"Your father is a wonderful gentleman," Charmaine told me. "And he's so brave. He's still so lucid after such a massive stroke. It's absolutely amazing."

I smiled. "Thanks. I know. He never gives up. He reads about the latest advances in stroke treatment and thinks some doctors might be able to make his left arm functional again. He even thinks he can drive again too. Even more than that, he expects to recover, work as a doctor, and help poor people in some third-world country." I shook my head.

Charmaine drew a sharp breath. "What incredible willpower."

"That's for sure. He had a huge amount of opposition from other scientists who didn't believe in his research, but he held his ground and never backed down. It paid off in the end, and I'm so glad his ideas have finally been accepted everywhere. A group of medical students visited him in the nursing home and told him how much they admired his work."

"And look how ill he is now. He lost his health trying to help others." She shook her head and pursed her lips.

I nodded. "His blood pressure went through the roof when he was only in his early fifties. He was already a walking time bomb, and it's only because of modern medicine that he's still alive."

"He was driven by a force beyond his control," Charmaine said with an air of clairsentience.

"In a way, he was. His mother was mercilessly ambitious, and she told me that when she was pregnant with Dad, she used to pray to God to give her another Hippocrates. Then, when she was pregnant again, she hoped for another boy and prayed that he would become a chemist. She pushed both of her boys to the limit with her impossibly high expectations. Well, my half uncle was never the academic type. He preferred business and was good at it, but he's very jealous of Dad. He often lies to strangers, pretending to have several university degrees and to be a retired chemist. He's never really accepted himself. It's pitiful."

Charmaine drew a sharp breath. "I know some mothers like that. They act as if they own their children and give them no peace. It's frightening what they do to their little souls."

"Oh, and I just remembered that my dad started off studying philosophy at the university. That was his first love, but his mother was furious. During his first year, when he came home to visit, a doctor who was an old friend of the family ridiculed him for studying philosophy. He called it nonsense and told him one can't make a living at being an expert in nonsense. He convinced him to switch to medicine. Mind you, he's still a philosopher in a way because he's in the research end of it."

"Talking about your dad, here he comes now," Charmaine said.

He stumbled on the rug as he approached us but managed to regain his balance before he fell. Charmaine and I rushed over to him and helped him navigate his way back to the living room. His left leg trembled, and he was gasping for air.

"I think it's time for me to take you back to the home now," I told him.

He didn't protest as I helped him put his jacket on. He looked dangerously pale.

"I look forward to seeing you again," he told Charmaine.

"Thank you, and the feeling is mutual," Charmaine said.

"See you when I get back?" I asked, giving Charmaine an intense look.

"I'll be here," she said.

On the way back to the nursing home, Dad told me he thought Charmaine was very intelligent, and he was impressed with her ability to converse about a great variety of topics.

When Dad was comfortably settled in his room, he held my hand and said, "I don't want to lose her yet. I've come to realize that family is much more important than ambition and achievement. That's what really counts in the end." His face twisted, as if he was going to cry.

I gulped, trying to dissolve the lump in my throat as a tear ran down my cheek. That was the first time he had told me that. He had finally realized that love was more important than anything else.

"I love you. Do you love me?" he asked with a thick voice.

"Yes. I love you, Dad," I whispered.

He pointed toward his cheek, expecting a kiss, and I leaned over and kissed him.

I was trembling in the car on the way back to the house. *They could both go at any time, and then I'll be all alone.* Then I told myself I couldn't afford to think like that because I had to stay strong and capable for everybody, and this was no time for a nervous breakdown.

Charmaine's car was still there when I got back.

After I walked into the house, I found her sitting at the dinette table and perusing her nurse's journal. "Your mom is okay, and she's been resting quietly. By the way, does your uncle know about your mom's situation?"

"Yes, he does. I called him yesterday. He's far away in Europe, though, so he's not much help."

"You know you can call me anytime if you need to talk. I'm only a few minutes away. Please, feel free to just pick up the phone. And my husband would love to help you too. In fact, he's a good handyman and can fix things around the house. If you need anything done, just let us know, and I'll send him over."

"Thanks! You have no idea how much that means to me."

"I have to go now, but I'll be back tomorrow at the same time." She got up. "I'll just check on your mom again before I go."

Mom was fine, and then I walked Charmaine to the front door.

"Remember, get her those B-complex vitamins," she said.

"See you tomorrow."

My uncle called me early in the morning, sounding quite excited. "Guess where I am?"

"In Europe somewhere?" I had no idea where he was.

"I'm in town, a few minutes from your house."

I was stunned. He used to live in Montreal and in Vancouver, but he hadn't been back to Canada in over forty years. I didn't know what to say.

"I stayed in a hotel last night and thought I'd surprise you in the morning."

"You sure have surprised me. Where exactly are you right now?"

"In downtown, close to the town hall. Can you pick me up?"

"Of ... of ... course," I said. "I'll ... I'll ... be right there in a few minutes."

I found him right away, we hugged, and then I drove him back to the house.

"I just had to come and see your mother when I heard how ill she was," he said. "You know how much I've always liked your mother."

I gave him a sideways glance.

"How are you?" he asked, smiling at me.

"Terribly tired, but I can't stop to rest. They're both so ill they need constant help." I sounded completely frazzled.

"Hmmm." He frowned.

Soon after I pulled into the garage, my uncle and I were in Mom's room.

Mom gasped when she saw my uncle. Her eyes were as wide as silver dollars.

"Hello! Surprised to see me?" my uncle asked, grinning at her.

Mom nodded but didn't smile.

"I flew with KLM to Amsterdam and then to Vancouver. You remember my old Vancouver friends? They drove me to the ferry in Horseshoe Bay, and then I took a taxi from Nanaimo. Not bad for a seventy-two-year-old man."

"How long do you plan to stay?" Mom still didn't smile at him, but he didn't seem to notice.

"A couple of weeks. I can stay here with you, can't I?" He looked hopeful.

"Yes, Dad's old room is right down the hall over there," I said as I pointed to it.

"Good! I'll put my things in there now and then come back to talk." He walked with the lively, purposeful energy of a boy about to go out for a bike ride.

While he was in the back room settling in, Mom whispered, "Why did he have to come here now? I'm too tired to handle him."

"We don't have a choice, do we?" I sighed long and hard.

Then the doorbell rang. I ran to the door and let Charmaine in. "You won't believe who just arrived," I said.

"Don't tell me it's your uncle." Her eyes widened.

"You guessed it. It will be a good distraction for us, especially for Dad," I said.

Charmaine met my uncle in the hall, and I introduced them before she checked in on Mom. "Your niece needs help looking after her parents," Charmaine said. "You came at the right time."

"Yes, I know," he said. "And I would like to see my brother today too." He gave me an expectant grin. "You can drive me to the nursing home today, can't you?"

"After I catch my breath, yes. And it's good that Charmaine is here to watch Mom."

I drove my uncle to see Dad a few minutes later. I was happy in one way but also resentful of having to take care of too many people at once. I wondered how long I would last.

"I can't wait to see the look on his face when he sees me," my uncle said with boyish glee as we approached the home. "I didn't call him to tell him anything."

"It might jumpstart his heart and cure him of his congestive heart failure," I said in a humorous tone of voice.

I knocked on Dad's door. "Yes, come in." He was very hoarse.

Dad was standing with his cane and trying not to wobble. He smiled at me and then exclaimed, "Oh! What? Ha! Ha! What are you doing here?"

"Surprise!" my uncle said, giving him a hug.

"Careful, he's not steady on his feet," I said. My arm shot out automatically toward Dad. It was good to see Dad's lopsided grin.

I left them alone to talk while I went down the hall to the nurse's station to tell them about my uncle's totally unexpected visit, and I had a dizzy spell on the way there. It was an unpleasant up and down feeling, as if the floor was rising up to meet my face. I began experiencing these spells while I was teaching, and an ear, nose, and throat specialist told me they were stress-related. He even ordered an MRI for my brain to make sure it was just stress, and the test was clear.

I thought back to the time when I looked after Dad at home for over three years after he had the massive stroke. The rehabilitation section of the hospital sent him home way too soon, and Mom's way of coping was to drink herself into oblivion. I thought back even further to when Dad was comatose in intensive care just after he had the stroke; after visiting him, I went back to our condo and found Mom on the floor behind the couch. There was a big, empty bottle of vodka sitting on the dining room table. A good friend was with me, and we stared at each other for a few seconds. Then we started laughing like kids and decided to go out for a drink ourselves.

Then I remembered my uncle and thought back to the summer afternoon in Porto Rafti on the east coast of Attica close to Athens when I was eight years old. We swam far away from the shore, and my uncle suddenly disappeared and let me flounder in the water, gasp for air, and struggle to get back to the shore. My grandparents were so far away they looked as tiny as fruit flies, and my parents were halfway around the world in Vancouver. I swam as hard as I could, looking down and hoping to see the sand and seeing only a profound blackness. I swam and swam and swam for dear life, and he didn't reappear until I stepped on the sandy shore. *What was he thinking? Maybe something like, "Surprise! I'm going to scare the living hell out of you, you little competitor for the family inheritance. Let's see how well you can swim all by yourself so far away from the safety of the shore."*

I wasn't surprised I was having dizzy spells. I was having them just trying to cope with my parents, and trying to cope with my uncle made me feel as if I were walking on the moon.

The nurses who were in the station told me that they were worried about me because I looked haggard and worn out. They said they had rarely seen anyone as dedicated and caring as I was, and they were amazed to see me visiting my dad day after day without fail. Many of the old folks had no visitors at all. They simply had been left to die at the hands of strangers. When they did pass away, all sorts of greedy, buzzard-like relatives would come out of the woodwork to fight for any money or property that was left over.

"I know I look worn out," I said. "My mom is supposed to die any day. There's a good nurse coming to the house, but it's not enough help because she can't stay very long, and my jumping bean of an uncle is here now. He wants to stay a while, and he's very demanding. I wouldn't mind checking into this home myself for a while to get a total break from everything." I looked at a room down the hall from the nurse's station. "Say, is that respite room available now?"

We all laughed. The respite rooms were for old folks.

One of the nurses looked at a calendar on her desk. "Actually, that respite room will be free tomorrow. Wanna grab it?"

We all laughed again.

Then it hit me. "Hey! Would you let my mom come here for a while? She really needs round-the-clock help and shouldn't have been sent home from the hospital in the first place. If she stays at home much longer, I'll end up in intensive care myself—in the zombie ward …"

"Great idea! Speak to the head nurse. She'll help you out." The nurses agreed on this.

I rushed to the head nurse's office, and she understood completely and made arrangements for my mom to be brought by transfer ambulance to the respite room. I thanked her over and over and over again. "You're a life saver," I told her.

"We're more than happy to help you out," she said. "Your mom will be in good hands. We have a happy hour once a week. We'll allow her to have a glass of wine, but that will be it. Her liver just might have a chance to recover. It's astounding how resilient the liver can be."

"Oh! You think there's hope for her!"

She nodded and gave me a slight, cautious smile.

Dad was very pleased to hear Mom would soon be a few steps down the hall from his room, and my uncle was amazed at how quickly the arrangements were made.

When my uncle and I arrived back at the house, I rushed to Mom's room to tell her and Charmaine that she'd be transferred to the nursing home the next day. Amazingly enough, Mom didn't protest, and I was glad she didn't have the strength to resist the paramedics.

"Guess what, Charmaine! The head nurse thinks Mom's liver may recover! Now I'm beginning to believe you when you tell me she's not dying!"

Charmaine gave me an omniscient smile and nodded as if to say, "I told you so."

My uncle went out for a walk, and I told Charmaine about my dad's comical reaction to my uncle's visit. She wanted to know every detail about their meeting.

I didn't want her to leave, as usual, but she said she'd be back to help Mom get ready for the transfer. She also reassured me that it was okay to call her anytime. In fact, she urged me to call anytime.

It was a full house the next morning as Charmaine, the paramedics, who thankfully arrived on time, and I did everything possible to place Mom on a stretcher and help her get comfortable. My uncle watched as we wheeled her out of her room, down the steps, and into the ambulance.

Charmaine left, and my uncle and I followed the ambulance to the nursing home.

Mom was wheeled straight to the respite room, and when she was settled, I told Dad. My uncle walked beside him and led him to the room so he could welcome her while I filled out more papers in the nurse's station. A nurse prepared some medications for Mom.

Thank God she's not protesting, and thank God I can sleep tonight knowing she's in the best place. The nurses already knew her quite well because they had seen her when she was visiting Dad before she ended up in the hospital. Everyone liked her, and that was another bonus.

I walked out of the big common activity room and onto the deck to admire the view of the fields and mountains. A couple of brown llamas were circling the pond, and hummingbirds with bright, fluorescent colors whirred around the suspended red plastic feeders. This was an ideal place for a terminally ill person. Dad would often say that the stunning view from his room was enough to wake up the dead.

My uncle joined me out on the deck and then wandered off to explore the lovely pastoral grounds. I checked in on Mom, who was resting, and then walked Dad back to his room.

When he finally sat down in the chair beside the big picture window, he sighed and said, "I don't know what I'm going to do about my brother. He wants me to give him a huge amount of money, saying he needs thousands and thousands of dollars to live and pay off his debts."

"Here we go again," I said and rolled my eyes.

"I told him I can't give him too much. I blamed you, saying I'm responsible for you because you didn't marry and have no one to look after you."

"Thanks," I said with a smirk.

"He asked me why you're not married and said you should have married long ago and been off my hands. He thinks you shouldn't have a claim to my money and says if it weren't for you and your mother, I'd be a lot more generous with him."

"Arrrgh!" I must have sounded like a hissing snake. "Sorry, Dad, but here I am, sacrificing my life as a caregiver for you and for Mom, and he dares to blame me and make these kinds of outrageous demands? What has he ever done for us except cause trouble? He *would* come here for the first time in forty years, now that you and Mom are too ill to refuse his demands."

Dad started trembling so much that his left leg bounced up and down like a needle in an industrial sewing machine. I was ready to give him his Dilantin to stop the seizure. Then he staggered to the bathroom, and I helped him pull his pants down as he plopped down on the toilet seat. He kept trembling and pulled the cord that was hanging on the wall. A care aide arrived and helped Dad get off the toilet.

My uncle appeared after Dad was comfortably stretched out on his bed.

I just glared at him, not knowing how I was going to keep my composure.

We said good-bye to my parents and headed out of the nursing home door toward the car.

When we were driving by the ocean close to the house, he said, "You're just a girl. I need your father's money more than you do. See if you can convince him to give me thirty thousand dollars."

"I have all these degrees and I'm just a girl? Ask him again yourself." I spoke with a firm and controlled tone of voice, but my face and neck felt as if I were trapped in a dry sauna set at 120 degrees Fahrenheit. *Now I see why some young people have fatal heart attacks. I'm going to have to talk to Charmaine before I end up in a cardiac ward.*

When my uncle was safely out of earshot, I called Charmaine and told her about the money drama and how angry I was to be told I'm "just a girl." *I've worked so much harder in my life than he ever has and I'm just a girl?* I wanted to scream loud enough to be heard in another country.

"I didn't want to say anything earlier because there was too much commotion and you were so preoccupied with everything.

However, the more I saw of your uncle, the more spooked I got. Just know that my husband and I are here for you, and it won't be too long before he goes back home. Don't let him upset you! I know that's easier said than done, but try. Just concentrate on your mother's recovery, and think of the good times you'll still have with her when she gets better."

"Thanks for your words of wisdom. I'll try to stay calm." *When pigs fly.*

My uncle left after a couple of weeks, promising to come back if the situation got worse. He said he wanted to take Dad back to the old country in an air ambulance and look after him there. He knew Dad wanted to go home to die. In reality, that would have given him the perfect opportunity to take full control of Dad's finances. He knew that Dad, being the older brother, felt responsible for him.

Mom stayed in the respite room for six weeks. Her abdomen shrank back to its normal size, and she realized she should just stick to a glass or two of wine a day. She was lucid, and her mood was much more positive than it had been in years. I was happy to bring her home in that condition. Dad was beautifully taken care of at the nursing home. Mom and I would break the monotony by frequently taking him out for lunch and bringing him home on weekends so he could sleep in his old bed and not feel abandoned.

Dad had suppressed his early interest in matters religious, mystical, and spiritual during his scientific career. He was so engrossed in the chemistry and biology of life that he saw all living things simply as interesting strings of molecules. He started out as a philosopher and thought the study of science would give him profound insights into the mystery of life. After a lifetime of research, he was no closer to the mystery than he was as a child. His science also didn't help him face the horrors of the unknown after he suffered a devastating stroke and congestive heart failure.

While he was still living at home, he read and admired

Foster Freed's articles in the "Pastor's Corner" section of our local newspaper and wanted to meet him. I took Dad to church one Easter Sunday, and the two men became instant friends. Foster visited Dad frequently after he was placed in the nursing home and helped him to see that religion and science are not necessarily incompatible. Foster worked very hard to convince Dad that he was a beloved child of God and that he didn't have to be a consistent winner in the academic rat race to earn that love. He asked him where those academic competitors and colleagues were and if they would have been able to help him face death. *That death that was hovering right outside the beautiful picture window, peering into the room, and waiting for the right moment to snatch him up.*

I went to the nursing home one sunny afternoon to visit Dad, and the head nurse beckoned to me in the hall beside her office. "Your dad doesn't have much longer," she whispered. "His lips are blue most of the time, and he has severe pitting edema in his legs. And he has a red rash on his abdomen, and that means his liver is failing."

I nodded slowly and frowned. "Thanks for telling me."

Foster was sitting by Dad's bed, and the two were busy talking away over the noise of the oxygen compressor machine, which sounded like a steam engine. Dad had two thin, clear plastic tubes in his nose.

I greeted them and sat down.

"Foster," my dad said with a burbly, hoarse voice, "did you know that your name means 'the one who brings light'?"

Foster looked delighted. "Thanks for telling me."

"That's a great name for you," I told him.

Foster laughed. "I'll leave you two alone now," he said as he got up. He waved at us and left.

I sat right next to Dad, who was stretched out flat on his back, and held his hand.

"I've been reading a Buddhist book on reincarnation, and Foster and I have been talking about life after death."

"Remember all that philosophy I read when I was a teenager? It was depressing, but it did tell me that science alone sure doesn't have all the answers."

"I love you," he whispered.

"I love you too, Dad."

"I always knew you'd be beside me, holding my hand at the end of my life." He smiled, and I almost bawled, as if he were already gone.

I sniffed the air around him. *What is that sickly sweet smell?* I had not smelled that in his room before. It was not a medication or anything like that. I sniffed again. It was Dad's body.

There were two cats living in the home, and the black-and-white one suddenly appeared at the foot of the bed. I had heard that those two cats would take turns staying with the patients who were very close to death. They would curl up on their beds. *Go away, kitty. Go away,* I thought.

I was too upset to stay for the rest of the afternoon, but I returned with Mom the next afternoon just after lunch. It was sunny, and the llamas were ambling around the pond. Dad was barely breathing through the tubes that delivered oxygen from the noisy compressor. His eyes were closed. "Do you know we're here?" I asked him.

"Yes," he said, sounding as if he were at the bottom of a well.

Mom and I sat with him for about an hour, and then Mom said, "I need to get out for a few minutes. We'll come back a little later."

When we got back, the social worker stopped us right beside the front door and told us that Dad had passed away.

"Oh my God!" I said.

The social worker gave me a long, tight hug. My face contorted in anguish as I looked up at the ceiling.

"I can't forgive myself for not being with him at the end!" Mom cried. "I just can't."

"That's almost always the way it happens," said the social worker.

"They wait for their loved ones to leave the room, and then they let their spirit go. Don't blame yourself." She tried hard to comfort us. Then I remembered a nurse who told me, "You're never prepared for the death of a loved one."

Another nurse said, "There was a beautiful light in the room when he took his last breath. He went toward the light."

Mom and I sat beside his body. The social worker and some of the nurses and care aides stayed with us for quite a while. He looked peaceful and content.

We found out that there were many angels in that nursing home who spent entire days and nights with Dad for the last few weeks of his life. They knew Mom and I were too exhausted to do that.

Foster gave Dad's eulogy and said that he had never worked with anyone who had such a terribly difficult time finding God and peace. Dad did find it just before he passed away, however, and apparently exclaimed, "I finally found God!" a few hours before the end. *How fascinating*, I thought as Foster gave the eulogy. Dad's family had saved a Jewish family from the Nazis during the war, and now Foster, an ethnic Jew who became a Christian minister, helped Dad find God so many years after the war. The favor was returned in the most profound possible way. Helping someone to die in peace is a gift beyond compare. Dad had learned to love and accept himself just minutes before his end.

I called Charmaine to tell her that Dad had passed away.

"Don't worry about your dad," she said with an enthusiastic tone. "I see him on the other side, and he's found a fellow spirit who's listening to him. She's helping him with the final stages of the healing of his soul. She knows he was not accepted for what he was when he was a child and that he was expected to become almost superhuman. His mother gave him no peace, starting with sexual abuse when he was little and continuing with threats of disinheritance when he was older. He buried himself in his books when he was a student, hoping to escape the torment in his soul. He became a workaholic. It was his self-medicating addiction. But the poison is leaving him now. He's happier … and … he'll continue to get happier …"

I was entranced. "Really? You really can see all that?"

"Clearly," she said.

"You were right about my mom, so I hope you're right about my dad."

She chuckled.

Charmaine, her husband, Mom, and I went out for dinner at a harborside restaurant a few weeks later. Charmaine's husband's mother was a healer, and he had inherited her ability to see auras around people's bodies. When Mom wasn't listening, he told me that her aura showed dark blue spikes shooting out of her head and upper body. That was not a good sign because dark blue colors, in his experience, meant disease. It could be disease of the body or of the spirit or both.

I wondered what was going on because Mom had recovered from her own near-death experience. Then it occurred to me that she must have been missing Dad. They had battled each other all their married life, but they were codependent and were so used to each other they actually missed each other when they were apart. That wasn't good to hear. I needed a break from all these crises. Grieving for Dad was all I could handle, and one cannot sidestep grief. One must simply go through it. Dad was a difficult person in many ways, but I was deeply attached to him. I was also in shock because it was the first time I had lost someone so close to me.

I called my uncle to tell him about Dad. He thanked me for telling him and then quietly sobbed.

A few days later, my uncle's lawyer called me and told me I had no right to my father's estate because some of it was inherited from my uncle's father and that he was contesting his father's will.

I got a similar call a few days after that. Then I changed my phone number and got caller ID. I never heard from my uncle or his lawyer again.

I called Charmaine and told her about the threats. "Change your name if necessary! Don't put up with any of this crap. You don't deserve it." Her voice was strong and clear and gave me courage.

Mom's physical health was fine, and that made it much easier for me to bear the grief of Dad's loss and the bitter realization that my uncle had become a permanent enemy.

Mom and I visited Dad's grave in the cremation garden every few days. It was a new garden, complete with young birch saplings, small pines, a fountain, and a pool. "I can't believe he's gone," Mom said one windy afternoon. She looked resigned and hopeless.

Dad passed away in the fall, and by spring, Mom was drinking heavily again. There was nothing anyone could do to stop her.

I came home one midmorning after grocery shopping and saw her in the kitchen. She was holding a long, sharp bread knife in her right hand and stabbed the air with it. "Don't move!" she shouted at me. "There's a monster sitting on your shoulder!" She lunged at me with the knife, her eyes wide with horrible fear.

I ran to the phone and called 911.

Two paramedics soon rushed into the kitchen and took the knife away from Mom. "Watch out! There are big black bugs crawling all over you. And they're all over the walls!" she shrieked at all of us.

When the paramedics heard about her health history and saw the big, almost-empty bottle of wine on the counter, one of them said, "She's probably got the DTs."

"DTs?" I asked, arching my eyebrows.

"Oh, sorry, that's the abbreviation for delirium tremens. That's what alcoholics sometimes get when they drink too much. They see creatures, especially black bugs, all over the place. We'll take her to the hospital. We just have to get her on the stretcher."

"Oh, yes, I've read about delirium tremens. That can be fatal." My heart fluttered.

They nodded, unfolded the stretcher, and moved Mom closer to it. "Ma'am, will you please lie down over here?" One of them placed a hand on the fresh white sheets on the stretcher.

"No! No!" Mom looked mortified. She screamed. "There's a monster sitting there! It looks like a gargoyle!"

"It's okay, Mom. There's no monster there." I put my arm around her shoulder. "Mom, it's okay. Please lie down so the nice men can take you to the hospital. You're not well."

It took about fifteen minutes before we could convince her to lie down. Even then, she looked frightened and disoriented.

I followed the ambulance to the hospital and stayed with Mom for hours in the emergency ward. At around 10:00 in the evening, an emergency room doctor told me, "Your mother is fine. You can take her home now. There's nothing we can really do for her."

"Take … take her home? She lunged at me with a bread knife." My jaw dropped in disbelief.

"She'll be fine now. Seniors have less resistance to alcohol, that's all," the doctor said with a shrug.

I couldn't convince the doctor to admit her and do further tests, so I was forced to take her out of the emergency ward and into the dark parking lot. I thought that was insane. Most people know that seeing black bugs and monsters is an indication of serious brain damage.

We left the hospital and stopped at an intersection about ten minutes later.

"That red light. It's a monster." Mom's voice was shaky, and her eyes were as wide as a screech owl's. She tried to open the car door and jump out.

I reached over her with my right arm and tried to calm her and keep the door shut. She kept on trying to jump out, and I tried to drive without killing us both in a head-on collision.

We made it home, partly because of long stretches of highway with no intersection lights.

Mom staggered to her bed and collapsed on it while I went to answer the phone. It must have rung at least fifteen times before I got to it; I could hear it even in the garage before I entered the house. *Who on earth would call at this time?*

"I'm so glad you're home! I had an awful feeling just after ten o'clock—a feeling that you were in terrible danger," Charmaine said quickly, with a breathy and agitated voice.

I explained everything to her and told her how right she was and how Mom had tried to jump out of the car. I told her I didn't know how I was going to make it through the night.

"Hang in there, and call us if anything happens during the night. Imagine sending her home, knowing that she had the DTs. Unbelievable."

I thanked her and braced myself for the onslaught of the night terror.

Mom got up around 3:00 a.m. and slammed doors so hard she nearly broke them. I thought a gang of burglars had broken into the house. I prayed for the stamina to survive until morning.

I called our family doctor first thing in the morning, and he came to our house. When he saw the catatonic condition we were both in, he said he'd arrange for a transfer ambulance to take Mom to the psychiatric ward at the hospital for a few days of rest and observation. There was no other way to deal with Mom, and I was immensely relieved that he could see that. When I asked about sending her to a detox center, he said that alcoholics have to sign themselves in, and no one can force them to do that. They are the only ones who can decide to check themselves in. I knew Mom would never do that. I wondered about those alcoholics whose brains were so damaged they could no longer make rational decisions.

I followed the ambulance as usual and accompanied Mom to the psychiatric ward. We waited for hours in the lobby area for a psychiatrist to interview her, and Mom tried to escape several times. I had to hold on to her with all the strength I could muster. She pulled on the glass doors every few minutes and nearly managed to escape from my grasp. I must have left deep marks on her arms.

When the psychiatrist finally arrived, she didn't want to hear about Mom's reasons for drinking and told me to go to Al-Anon and get counseling for myself. I was stunned. At least she filled out the necessary paperwork and took Mom to the nurse's station. The nurses tried to settle her down and finally managed to sedate her enough so she wouldn't try to escape.

I was so relieved to go home and have some peace by myself for a change.

The phone rang at midnight. *What now? A phone call from Dracula?*

The nurses were on the phone, saying that Mom wouldn't stay in her bed. She was lying down and crying on the floor beside the bed. They didn't know what to do with her and were begging me to come and get her.

"Come and get her? Come and get her? You must be kidding," I said in a very stubborn tone. "You're working as a team over there, and I'm all alone and I should handle her here all by myself? Sorry, I'm not coming. And don't try to send her home in an ambulance, because I won't answer the door. I won't let her in. I need a break."

"Will you come and visit her in the morning at least?" the nurse on the phone asked, sounding very nervous.

"Of course." *What a way to feel wanted.*

When I arrived in the psychiatric ward in the morning, the nurses told me Mom had been moved to a private room. The door had a large, clear, plastic observation bubble at eye level. She was on her side, resting on the bed and facing the far wall. *God help us.*

I opened the door slowly and walked toward her. "Mom? Mom?" I walked around the bed to face her.

She opened her eyes and looked at me with that familiar look of terror.

"How are you?" I asked, stroking her hair.

"Don't leave me here all alone," she said.

"I won't. I won't."

"I can't believe he's gone," she muttered in a dejected tone, as if Dad had abandoned her on purpose.

"I can't either, but it's a miracle he lasted as long as he did, and so many wonderful people helped to look after him. We have to think of that. And what kind of a life was that for him, being brain damaged, crippled, and incontinent for five and a half years?" I put my arm around her shoulders.

"He didn't love me," she mumbled.

"Yes, he did. He said so when I brought him home, don't you remember? He really meant it too. He told me he wasn't ready to lose you." I sounded soothing and affectionate.

"Mmph," she sighed. "I want to come home." She closed her eyes, as if she were praying.

I walked to the nurse's station. "How long will she stay here? Do you know?"

"A day or two at the most. We can't keep her here much longer."

"I can't take her home yet. She's too much for me right now. Isn't there a place she could go from here for a couple of weeks before I take her home?" I asked, sounding like I wasn't going to back down.

"You could try a private nursing home. Maybe the social worker can help you."

I walked to the social worker's office and told her about the situation.

"Here's the phone book. There are some private nursing homes in there," she chirped. She looked like a nice person but didn't seem to be used to dealing with real emergencies.

"I'll try to find one, but I'm concerned about getting her over there. Knowing her, she'll probably refuse to go. She wants to come home!"

"I can arrange for a transfer ambulance." She was still calm, as if she had no idea what a crisis this really was for Mom and me.

"Thanks, and can I use your desk phone?" I asked, speaking quickly.

She turned it around, and I tried several numbers. No one had space.

Then I remembered seeing a van with the name and number of a private lodge. I found the name in the book and called. *Please, please, have a space for Mom. You're my only hope.*

The owner of the lodge answered and said she had only one room left for a two-week stay and that I would have to secure it with a deposit as soon as possible. I ran out of the hospital, drove to the home, and made the deposit just in time. Another person was right behind me and would have grabbed the room if I hadn't rushed like a madwoman.

I felt Mom would be happy there. The owner seemed really nice and had furnished and decorated the lodge beautifully. She seemed to care about her residents.

Charmaine called just after I got home. She sensed that there was another crisis with Mom.

"She'll be transferred to a private home for a couple of weeks, but what happens after that? Mom will never check herself into a detox center."

"What silly laws we have!" Charmaine sighed heavily. "Even in Washington State an alcoholic can be signed into a detox center by family or friends."

"I just hope Mom will improve before she comes home."

"She will. You'll still have some good times together. Wait and see." Her tone was so warm and confident that I believed her.

"You're so compassionate. You're like the sister I never had," I told her after we discussed my predicament for over two hours.

"I had two wonderful brothers, but I always wanted a younger sister," Charmaine said with a sincere longing in her voice. "Maybe you're that sister. It's no accident that we met, you know."

"I agree. It was no accident. You literally walked into my life through the front door just at the right time and helped me cope with all these crises. I don't know what I would have done without you."

Charmaine gave a light chuckle. "I've helped a lot of people over the years, and I'm more than happy to do it for you." Then her voice lowered and softened. "I've even helped some desperate souls who had already died and were stuck in a kind of a hellish twilight zone."

I gasped. "What?"

"Oh, yes. I visited Europe with my husband when I was much younger, and when we were touring close to one of the notorious Nazi death camps, I was overwhelmed by an incredibly strong feeling—a feeling that insisted that I actually walk into one of the prison areas. Not just the administration area but a prison area! My husband and his relatives were mortified and didn't want me to go in there, but I was drawn to it, as if aliens were sucking me into a UFO."

"Good God," I whispered.

"Well, I went in quite far by myself and then stopped short when I felt the strong presence of three souls crying out for help. I actually felt a pressure on my shoulders, as if they were touching me. I suddenly knew what was wrong with them! They couldn't find peace because they didn't know the war was over. I told them what year it was and that the war had ended decades ago. I told them they could go away in peace now. They were still in terrible anguish, but I kept repeating that the war was over and that they were free to go. Then I felt an incredible collective relief. I felt that they finally believed me, so I started walking back to the entrance. When I arrived at the door, I looked back and saw their faces! They had followed me out of the torture area and then vanished at the outside door. I know they entered a peaceful plane on the other side."

"Imagine, helping desperate souls like them. You're amazing."

"Yes, they sometimes communicate with sensitives like me. I'm like a channel, a conduit of sorts. It's exhausting to be a sensitive, but what can I do? I was born this way."

"I'll bet you've had out-of-body experiences too," I said.

"Very much so! When I was a young nursing student, I was walking back to the hospital in Los Angeles after lunch one afternoon when I felt like I'd been zapped by a strong current. The hairs on the back of my neck stiffened, and my skin felt like it was burning. I knew my fiancé was in trouble. I just knew it. Then I had an out-of-body experience. I actually arrived in Hawaii, where he was studying, and slid into the car he was driving. I sat beside him as he died in a horrific head-on collision. I held his head in my hands, cried, and said good-bye to him. Then I arrived back at the hospital doors, all wet and shaking violently. A few days later, I was notified that my fiancé had been killed in a terrible car accident at the exact time I had the experience." She was out of breath, and I was spellbound.

"You're like the psychics the cops use to find missing people and all that. Probably even more gifted. Have you ever done that?"

"No, sweetie, no. I don't use my gift professionally."

A couple of months after Mom came home from the private nursing home, I took her out for lunch at a golf club restaurant. She was smartly dressed, had a lovely hairdo, and looked dignified. We sat on the patio under an umbrella and admired the potted flowers, the birds, the fountain in the pond, the fairways, the trees, and the jagged mountain in the distance.

Charmaine and her husband appeared as we were finishing our meal. "How good to see you," she said. "Isn't this a beautiful place? We love to come here and admire the view."

They stopped to talk for a few minutes. Charmaine had a mysterious smile on her face that puzzled me until I remembered her prediction about Mom. She had seen her as being well dressed and dignified and being in a beautiful place just like this at a time when almost everyone else had given up on her.

Mom and I did have some good times together for several years after that. She always wanted someone to tell her story, and she was still lucid when *Banished from the Homeland* was published. People loved her for being so courageous, and that warmed her heart.

She lived for seven years after Charmaine helped her recover from liver failure.

Those seven years (and the many years before that) probably would have been much more enjoyable for her and for me if she had sought professional help for her damaged self-esteem, war-induced PTSD (it is apparently common for refugees like my mother to experience an intensification of PTSD symptoms as they age), depression, and anxiety. She may not have had to self-medicate with alcohol to obliterate the smoldering pain in her soul, and that would have made my dad's life infinitely easier as well.

But she was too proud to seek the help she needed; she thought she could conquer her anxiety on her own by drinking herself into oblivion, and it didn't seem to occur to her that she had dragged my father and me down with her. She, like so many others, didn't realize that there is no longer any shame in getting help to improve one's mental health. One can improve one's own life and the lives of one's loved ones and friends by doing so. Gone are the days of laying down on a psychiatrist's couch for a minimum of three years; one can often get valuable, life-changing help in just a few months. Sometimes a few weeks can make all the difference between prolonged misery and emotional relief.

If I would have known how vital it is to have strong boundaries, I might have looked after myself more and not neglected my own needs almost to the point of self-destruction. Mom and I had become codependent, and I was so obsessed with caregiving for both parents that I had no time to learn to love and accept myself. On the contrary, I sometimes wondered if I was doing enough for them, and I even felt guilty about placing them in nursing homes when their health worsened. I also felt inadequate and frustrated because I gave up teaching to become a full-time caregiver and wasn't earning a regular salary. I sometimes wondered why I bothered to get a string of university degrees if I wasn't going to use them.

Mom had to flee her beloved homeland because of a cruel dictator, and Dad and I suffered along with her as secondary casualties of Stalin. If mankind evolves to a point where people love and accept each other so much that they no longer send each other to labor camps and force each other into exile, life on earth will be just a little bit more like it is in heaven.

Chapter 17

Karma

Vito and I strolled around the campus's art museum one midspring Saturday morning and admired the painted Japanese screens and bronze statuettes of Hindu gods and goddesses. We were both grateful that the dirty snow was almost gone and that we could take a break from our studies to enjoy the campus grounds.

"Which god is that?" I asked Vito as I pointed to a statuette of a handsome young man. I assumed Vito would know because he had just finished a course in eastern art. He was completing a degree in biomedical engineering, but he was interested in everything.

"That's Shiva, the destroyer," Vito said. "He's the ultimate destroyer of the ego and of the universe."

"Brrr." I shivered. "We've grown up with the fear of a nuclear holocaust, so I believe there are gods of destruction out there." I stared at the statue for at least a minute.

"You have the most intense eyes I have ever seen. They project an incredible inner strength," Vito said with a profoundly respectful tone. "In fact, I've never seen such eyes, not even in a man. And not only that, but you also exude a Christ-like compassion." He gave me an affectionate half smile.

"Wow. I'm ... I'm stunned that you can see right through me. And what a compliment! Thanks for telling me. No one has ever praised me that much." I felt fabulous.

We ambled out of the museum and sat on a stone bench by a pond surrounded by pink and yellow flowers. It was so relaxing to feel the sunrays and watch the flowers quivering in the breeze.

"Let me take some pictures of you," Vito said as he got up and took a camera out of his jacket pocket. "I'm taking a photography course, and I want to impress my prof."

I giggled. "You're sure you want *me* in a picture if you want to impress your prof? Why don't you just take some pictures of the flowers and the museum? It looks like a little Greek temple."

Vito laughed. "No, no ... I'll take some pictures of you and the flowers."

I got up, stood at the edge of the pond, and tried to look natural.

Vito took several pictures, and then we headed back to the campus dorms.

We met in the cafeteria at lunchtime a few days later. "Now that one should impress your prof," I said as I admired one of the pictures he showed me. My face was surrounded by flower petals, making it look like the center of a colorful daisy.

Vito smiled. "I superimposed a flower picture over the close-up of your face. I didn't think it would work, but it did. I had fun doing that."

"Could I have a copy of this one? It's unique."

"Of course. And by the way, there's a dance at my dorm at nine o'clock this Friday night. I hope you can make it. And tell your other friends."

* * * * *

My friends and I could hear the loud disco music emanating from Vito's dorm long before we got there. We all laughed when we managed to squeeze ourselves through the crowd at the door. "Look at Vito," one man chortled. "He's dancing like an elephant in heat."

"Yeah, look at him," another man said as he sipped beer from a plastic cup. Vito, smiling as if he had just reached nirvana, was entertaining us by gyrating in the middle of the dance floor.

When the music stopped, Vito saw me and beckoned to me.

I walked over to him and thanked him for putting on such a show. Beads of sweat rolled down his forehead. He took his glasses off and wiped the lenses, and we sat down by a window.

"I needed to dance to let off some steam," he said. "I broke up with my girlfriend earlier today."

"You're kidding! I saw you holding hands with her about three weeks ago," I said.

"My parents phoned and told me they didn't approve of her. They threatened to disown me in every way if I continued to see her," he said with a weak, listless voice.

"How horrible." I patted him on the shoulder.

"Thanks for listening. You're such a good friend," he said. Now his eyes looked vacant, as if the vibrant spirit of life had just flown out of his body.

I wondered how he could dance with such passion one minute and then be so lifeless the next minute. He didn't dance for the rest of the evening, even though some other friends and I tried to coax him back onto the dance floor.

I saw Vito in the noisy, crowded cafeteria at breakfast the next morning and walked over to him with my tray. "How are you feeling this morning?" I asked as I sat down across from him.

"Not too good," he said with a hoarse voice, his face unshaven.

"I've got a funny story for you," I said. "You've been all over the world, so you might appreciate this." I told him about a shop at the airport in Zurich. The walls were covered from floor to ceiling with cuckoo clocks, and they were all whirring, buzzing, clicking, and cuckooing at the same time. I tried to imitate the pandemonium of sounds and jerky movements as if I were a stand-up comedienne.

His vacant expression gradually morphed into one of boyish amusement, and he gave me a toothy smile. "Thanks. That's just what I needed. Something ridiculous and surreal."

"Anytime," I said with a cat that just swallowed a canary smile.

"By the way, I do have a copy of that picture for you," he said as he took his wallet out of his pocket. "And my prof really was impressed with it." He took it out of the wallet and gave it to me.

"Thanks so much. I'm going to put this one in an album."

"As you know, I'm graduating next month, and I've already got a job. Make sure you give me your home phone number before I leave. I like to keep in touch with my friends."

"Of course. And congratulations and good luck. Maybe you'll find a new girlfriend soon—one your parents will like."

"I hope so. In any case, I'll be calling you."

On the day before he left, Vito came to my dorm room to say good-bye. He gave me the warmest, sweetest, friendliest hug I had ever received from anyone.

After I graduated, I moved back home and looked for a job.

Vito called me and told me he was happy at work but that he had been disowned by his parents because he had married a woman they couldn't stand. Even his brothers had turned against him. He was often overcome by terrible rages that drove him to kick and punch furniture.

He called me long-distance for several years and was always as friendly as he was in our student days. Even if we talked for two hours, he said it was his pleasure to pay because his friends meant everything to him. His rages continued, however, and he told me how much he hated several members of his family and that he wouldn't speak to them at all.

One day Vito suddenly stopped calling, and I couldn't reach him no matter how hard I tried, so I eventually gave up on him.

I came home one Sunday afternoon after visiting my mom in the hospital's psychiatric ward; I was terribly restless and wondered what I could do to calm down. I knew I could call Charmaine, but I didn't want to be a pest by calling her too often.

The phone rang. I wondered if Charmaine had read my mind.

"Hi, my old friend, this is Vito." He sounded calm and very friendly.

"Vito! What a nice surprise! You have no idea how good it is to hear your voice. You called just at the right time. My mom is in the psych ward, and I think I'm going crazy myself," I said, speaking rapidly.

"Sorry I disappeared for so long. And I'm sorry to hear about your mother."

"How are you? Where are you?"

"I'm in Toronto. I had a nervous breakdown a couple of years ago, and I have heart trouble. I often have panic attacks that are so bad I end up in the emergency room." He still sounded calm.

I gasped sharply. "How awful."

"The psychiatrist who helped me recover from my breakdown told me I've never recovered from the sexual abuse I endured as a boy. I wasn't actually raped, but my soul felt raped."

"Oh my God, Vito." I was thunderstruck. "You never told me any of this before. It's amazing that you managed to study so hard and get such a good engineering job. Does your wife know about all this?"

"She knows, and luckily, she's very empathic. By the way, we're divorced, but she's still my best friend. Actually, she's the best friend I've ever had."

"Really? Hmmm." I didn't know what to think about that.

We talked for over two hours, discussing every aspect of our lives. He felt very sorry for my mom and for me. He promised to call again soon and gave me his number as well. I was grateful that he had reappeared in my life when I needed all the support I could get.

Vito called me frequently, helping me cope with Mom's instability. I was always stimulated by his conversation and continued to be amazed by his determination to succeed in life. He told me how much he valued our old friendship and that he never wanted to lose touch with me again.

A couple of years after Mom recovered from her mental breakdown, Vito visited us. He stayed in a waterfront hotel for a few days, and we enjoyed showing him around. He treated Mom with great respect and tenderness, and she thought he was very intelligent and sophisticated.

Soon after he went back home, he called and invited me to visit him. However, he also said that his ex-wife was thinking about moving back in with him and that he wouldn't speak to me if I called while she was with him.

I made the travel arrangements to visit him but cancelled them a few days later because I felt that he was playing cat and mouse games with me. His words, "I won't talk to you if you call when she's here" invaded my mind like vicious nanoparticles injected by an alien brain surgeon.

"I won't come to visit you after all," I said in a firm tone when I called him. "A real friend would not threaten to cut me off like that."

"Oh, please, please come. You mean a lot to me. Actually, I

treasure you!" He sounded so sincere and so convincing that I reversed the cancellation and reinstated my trip plans.

"Wonderful. I can't wait to see you," he said when he found out I was really coming.

I arrived in the hotel one lovely July morning, checked in, unpacked, and ran down to the pool to relax. Vito had left a message saying he would pick me up after he finished work and would take me out for dinner. I was really excited and couldn't wait to see him again. I hoped that his confusion would work in my favor and that he would realize how wrong he had been to threaten to cut me off.

The phone rang in my room just after I finished my swim. "Hello?" I was breathless.

"Hi." Vito's voice was cold and mysterious. "I'm going to be a little late because my ex-wife says she wants to discuss the possibility of moving back in with me. But if she decides to move back in, I won't be able to pick you up as planned."

"Oh ... Oh ... really." I was breathless, feeling as if he had whacked me in the stomach with the thick end of a baseball bat. I knew we were just friends and that he had every right to welcome his ex-wife back into his life, but I was romantically attracted to him. My feelings for him had deepened just as he kissed me on the cheek before flying back home after his visit. I was still grieving Dad's loss and trying to recover from endless, grueling years of around-the-clock caregiving. I had lost a lot of my youthful stamina, and my personal boundaries were too porous. I felt uncharacteristically weak and vulnerable. The red flags of his vacillating behavior were there, but I chose to ignore them.

"I'll call you around five o'clock in any case," he said.

"Fine," I said in a steady voice, not wanting him to guess how disappointed I was.

He called later to tell me he wouldn't be able to take me out for dinner but that he would take a day off of work the next day to show me around the city and spend the entire day with me. *How bittersweet.*

I wore a new pair of decorated blue jeans and a navy velour top, sat on a bench, and waited for Vito in the hotel lobby. He appeared at the front doors on time, wearing casual clothes and looking rather professorial. I got up and walked toward him, and he greeted me with a casual nod. I smiled as he opened the passenger door of the car for me, but he didn't smile at me.

After he sat down behind the wheel, he gave me an accusatory glance. It was as if he resented me for visiting him and perhaps adding to the confusion in his life. That burning look in his eyes only lasted a couple of seconds, but it was frightfully sinister.

He warmed up to me when we were a few blocks away from the hotel. "I'm so glad you're here. I'm sorry about last night. I really wanted to see you."

"You did?" I arched an eyebrow and gave him a suspicious sideways glance.

"Yes, very much. My ex-wife won't be moving back in with me after all."

"Why not?"

"She says she wants to be independent." He looked dejected.

"She may change her mind again," I said. *What the hell is going on between them?*

As we approached a bridge, Vito drew a sharp breath.

I turned my head to get a better look at him. "Are you okay?"

He didn't answer right away. He cleared his throat and then spoke. "I was driving over this bridge a couple of years ago while I was so depressed I wanted to commit suicide."

I gasped.

"I wanted to crash right through the railing."

"Good God," I whispered.

"I nearly did it, but I could hear a strong voice urging me not to do it. There was a presence in the car with me. I don't know who or what it was, but it was a presence."

"Talk about getting help from the other side," I said. "That's amazing."

Vito nodded. "I tried to commit suicide the same way a few months later, and the same strong presence commanded me not to do it."

I felt terribly sorry for him. "It's too bad you chose this route today. Maybe you shouldn't have driven over this bridge. All those awful memories are too much."

He glanced down at my breasts, his eyes lingering there for a few seconds. "I'm having heart palpitations, so we'll drive a little more, then we'll go for lunch, and then I'll take you back to your hotel. I'll have to go home to take my medication."

"Oh, you're on medication?" I was very concerned.

He nodded. "It stabilizes my heart and helps me cope with panic attacks. A friend sometimes drives me to the hospital when I have severe attacks."

I wondered how someone so intelligent, so educated, so successful, and so well-travelled could be so pitifully unstable. Then I remembered what he told me about the sexual abuse. In spite of that, I was attracted to him and wanted to help him recover. At a deeper level I knew he was wrong for me and that he had caused me a lot of pain, but I couldn't help myself.

"I wish I could help you feel better," I said affectionately.

"Thanks. You and your mother, you both fly toward the light. You're positive, cheerful souls. I wish I could be like that, but I'm not. I've always flown toward the darkness."

"You have?" I asked, frowning.

"Yes, and I envy the ones who live in the light."

We had lunch in a casual bistro. The food was excellent, but we hardly talked. Vito checked his watch frequently, as if he couldn't wait to get rid of me. I wondered why he had asked me to visit him in the first place and if he really was as ill as he said he was. I wondered why he told me he treasured me. *I treasure you, I treasure you, I treasure you.* The nanoparticles took charge of my brain again. *You mean a lot to me, you mean a lot to me, you mean a lot to me. I won't talk to you, I won't talk to you, I won't talk to you.*

Vito drove me back to the hotel and told me to continue sightseeing on my own.

I saw him a couple of more times during my visit. He made tea for me in his apartment, but he was cool and distant—so cool, in fact, that I felt guilty for visiting him. I felt like an unwelcome guest.

I was glad to get home.

He called me a few days later. "I miss you already." He sounded desperate. "You're so kind and humorous. You cheer me up."

"I do?"

"Very much. And I'm sorry I was cool toward you in my apartment. I was thinking about my wife, wondering where she was going to go next."

"Really."

"I wanted to sit beside you on the sofa and hold your hand, but I didn't because I couldn't stop thinking about her." He spoke the words "hold your hand" with great tenderness.

I was silent. *You wanted to sit beside me and hold my hand. So why didn't you?*

"One of these days I'd like to visit you again," he said in a loving tone.

He sent me affectionate e-mails and phoned to tell me he missed me.

He visited me the next summer. Mom was in a nursing home, so he stayed in my house. We visited Mom, who was still somewhat lucid, and she enjoyed seeing him.

I drove Vito to one of the most beautiful beaches in the area one warm morning, and we sat in the car to enjoy the view. *This is life-giving, life-affirming scenery. Who wouldn't be ecstatic looking at that white, seagull-packed sandbar, the sparkling ocean, and the distant glaciers on the mainland? Surely Vito will want to fly out of the darkness and toward the light now.*

He gazed at the view and then turned his head to look at me. "Something about you still haunts me," he said, sounding conspiratorial and looking very serious.

I knitted my brows and waited.

"You cancelled your trip last year. You said you'd come to see me, and then you changed your mind." His voice was low and steady.

"I cancelled it because you told me you wouldn't talk to me, but I came anyway, didn't I?"

"Yes, you did." He put his warm hand over mine.

I enjoyed his touch but not his attempt to make me feel guilty. I squirmed inside.

That evening, as we were relaxing on a loveseat in the family room, Vito asked me if he could massage my shoulders. I agreed.

"May I kiss you?" His voice was soft and affectionate.

I turned my face toward him, and we kissed and hugged for a long time.

"You have a strong body," I said as I ran my fingers over his arms and chest.

"No, I don't. It's just flab." He sounded sarcastic and impatient, as if he hated himself.

We hugged and kissed all night.

"I wish I wouldn't have to leave," he said in the morning.

"I wish you wouldn't have to either," I said with a sigh.

"I wish I could take you back home with me," he said with a sincere voice.

"You do?" I grinned at him. I was thrilled to hear him say that.

We had a quick, light breakfast, and then the cab arrived to take him to the airport.

"I had a fantastic time. Thanks, and I'll call you when I get home," he said.

"Yes, do call and tell me how the flight was," I said.

I visited Mom right after Vito left and took her out of the nursing home for a drive. She was glad to hear that Vito had a fantastic time.

After I got back to the house, the phone rang. I wondered if Vito was calling me from the airport.

"Hi, it's Charmaine! Are you okay?" She spoke rapidly, sounding terribly concerned.

"Hi, Charmaine. It's good to hear your voice. Yes, I'm okay. That friend I told you about—Vito—he was here for a few days, and he just left. I didn't call you because I was too busy driving him all over the place."

"Are you absolutely sure you're okay?"

"I think so."

"You were in terrible danger last night. There was an angry, explosive presence in your house all night, an almost evil presence that wanted to erupt and harm you in a big way, but luckily for you, there was a protective angel there as well. I'm not kidding. I was praying for you all last night." She was just as confident about her perception as she was when she told me my mom was going to live.

"Th... thanks for telling me. Now you've really got me wondering what's going on."

"Always call me if you're in danger, even if it's in the middle of the night. My husband and I will be there for you." The urgency was still in her voice.

"I ... I will. And thanks for your concern."

Vito called me in the evening. "I got home, and I miss you already. I miss your kisses."

"I miss you too," I said.

It was a very short conversation.

He called a few days later in the evening.

"I don't want you in my life! How dare you try to get close to me!" he shouted, telling me I was an unwelcome invader in his life. I tried to protest, but I couldn't interrupt the diarrhea of hateful words. I couldn't believe this was the same person who wanted to take me back home with him. When he finished, he slammed the phone down.

I immediately dialed his number, but I only got his voice mail. I tried again, but I didn't leave a message. I sat by the phone for a long time, trying to understand and accept what had happened.

I didn't sleep at all that night, and called Charmaine early in the morning.

She was terribly upset and sorry for me but not surprised. "It was karma. I feel that you were paying for something an ancestor did. It was beyond your control. But you're going to be okay. He's a very dangerous man, and I know you feel awful, but you're going to be okay."

"God, I hope so."

I felt an overwhelming need to consult a psychologist, and I called one right after I spoke with Charmaine. He answered right away and told me to go to his office, which was in his house, in the late afternoon. He lived quite close to me, and I fully explained my reasons for being there when we were alone in his office. He congratulated me for having a strong instinct of self-preservation and said, "Some people get counseling after being touched by a feather, and others get it only after being hit by a dump truck."

He laughed when I said that Vito was my "dump truck," and

then he told me that Vito seemed to be the type of person who enjoys wallowing in misery. He felt that Vito could have developed a much more positive attitude toward life if he would have had proper counseling and would have tried hard to lift himself out of the mud. Most of us can recover from all kinds of abuse if we learn to change the way we think about it. When we realize we didn't deserve the abuse and that we have the cure in our own hearts, we can start on the path toward self-love and self-acceptance. Then we will attract more positive people and circumstances and will send light into other people's lives as well. Most of us need all the light we can get.

The psychologist, who had also taught at a prestigious university, was an expert in the field of energy psychology and helped me release years of volcanic stress in just a few weeks. He used the colorful expression, "Shit rolls downhill" to illustrate the domino effect of abuse. We tend to be attracted to what we're familiar with until we get the kind of help that can heal us. Then we can sidestep the juggernaut and watch it roll by. It felt wonderful to be told that I was an amazing person. The psychologist resonated with every aspect of my being and told me the healing work we did would keep filtering through me long after the sessions were over. He hoped I would learn to love my own company so much that I would feel perfectly content and complete whether there was a significant other in my life or not.

Whenever Charmaine called me, she would bolster my self-esteem and confirm what the psychologist said. She wanted me to reach a highly evolved level of spiritual completeness and insisted that I was doing fine by myself, even though I didn't always feel that way. We agreed that it was better to live alone than to be in a negative and soul-destroying relationship.

I thought back to the time Vito and I admired the statue of Shiva the destroyer in the art museum. The destruction or deconstruction of my old life and my outdated ways of thinking was necessary so that a newer, fresher life could flourish. I longed to become the person the psychologist and Charmaine said I was: a radiant being with a great attitude.

Part III

Chapter 18

Full of Hope

After I stared hard into my past and understood why it had been unnatural at first for me to say, "I love you" to myself, I came back to the present with an intense desire to survive and enjoy every second of my life. I had been judged mercilessly by so many people, but the negative projections of their own misery no longer had a grip on me because I realized I had not deserved one iota of it. *They* were the ones with the problem, *not me*.

Most of the cynical, demonic voices had flown out of my brain. I could laugh at the schoolyard bullies; the racial prejudice; the rigid classification of the track tests; my family's rejection of my talents; men telling me I didn't have movie-star looks, a strong character, or a true passion for music; people telling me I was too proud and selfish and deserved to be gang-raped; others calling me an "older woman"; and my uncle telling me I was "just a girl." I no longer wanted to punish myself for giving up regular salaried work and looking after my parents for so many years. I did what I had to do, and I could love myself all the more for having such a self-sacrificing and altruistic soul. The caregiving, as strenuous as it was, still gave me enough free time to create my own style of music and to begin writing some of the stories I had longed to write. I was grateful for my new life, no longer had regrets about the past, and was full of hope for the future.

I was very pleased with myself for having the courage to delve into my turbulent past while undergoing chemo, and that seemed to give me extra energy and stamina. I only needed a few painkillers and some sleeping pills during the four weeks after my first round of chemo. The dreaded nausea never came, partly due to new and improved antinausea medications that happened to be effective in my case. I kept walking and swimming and rarely needed an afternoon nap. Dr. A told me he thought I was going to be okay during the second and third rounds, and that was music to my ears.

I called N, a lady who owned a nursing home and who had looked after my mother for a couple of weeks after she came out of the hospital. She was shocked to hear about my illness and scolded me for not calling her sooner. She wanted to pick me up after the second round of chemo and take me back to her place for the night.

The October morning when I had the second round of chemo, the routine was the same as the first one; I was given the antinausea IV for half an hour, followed by chemo for about four hours. The nurses were as warm and friendly as ever, and so were the volunteers, who offered me cupcakes, magazines, juice, and water. As before, there were at least six or seven other patients sitting in the large, comfortable chairs next to mine. Once again, I experienced the muscle tension that made me want to jump out of the chair and pace around the room. I kept shifting, watching the clock, and wondering when the torture would end. At least it was easier this time, because I knew I was not allergic to the antinausea drug or to the carboplatin and paclitaxel, which were the chemo drugs.

N picked me up after the session at around 2:00 in the afternoon, and she told me she was having a Baha'i study group coming over for dinner and discussion at around 6:00. She hoped I would be up to joining the group after an afternoon nap.

The nap was refreshing, and there were at least eight people in the living room when I came downstairs. A handsome, middle-aged gentleman was introduced as the famous Baha'i architect who had designed the Lotus temple in New Delhi; it is apparently the most frequented building in the world. His stunningly beautiful young daughter and her handsome young husband were also there. N introduced me and told them about my ordeal and how I was brave and hopeful in spite of it. The daughter exclaimed, "I had an amazing dream a few nights ago! I saw a woman who had cancer but who was full of hope."

"Wow. My hope really must be very strong if it even reaches the minds of total strangers. That's incredible," I said as I sat down close to her.

The family then shared that the beloved wife of the architect had recently died of cancer.

After a tasty, spicy buffet dinner, N distributed Baha'i workbooks and pencils, and we all settled comfortably in the living room. The architect thumbed through his Baha'i prayer book, and said, "I would like to read the healing prayer for this lady." Someone gave me a copy of the book, and I read along with him silently. It was a very moving prayer, beseeching God to take the sick woman beneath the shadow of his tree of healing and give her tranquility, healing, and protection. I thanked him when he finished reading, and he smiled sweetly. I could feel myself becoming more and more spiritual by the minute. C had introduced me to Buddhism, I went to my own church, and now I was in a Baha'i study group. I had neglected the spiritual side of myself for years, and I began to see what I had been missing for so long; I felt a deep yearning for spiritual development.

A couple of days after I got home, I looked at my abdomen above my waist and saw an unusual bulge. *Oh my God, it's come back. That wasn't there before.* I feared I would have a panic attack. By the evening, I couldn't stand it anymore and called the after-hours number for cancer emergencies. I got a doctor in Victoria, who was very polite and sounded really confident and knowledgeable; he thought it must have been simply a structural change caused by the hysterectomy. He told me that my organs must have shifted around and said it was too soon for a recurrence. However, he urged me to get it checked out as soon as possible at the clinic.

Charmaine called me soon after I hung up to tell me she could feel that I was terribly worried. She tried to calm me down by assuring me that nothing was wrong. While we were talking, she suddenly had a vision about my future: "I see you really, really happy! I see your sparkly name dancing around in the air, like it's saying, 'This is my time now, wheee, yippee!' This is your time, girl. The rest of your life is going to be all about you, and you're going to enjoy yourself more than ever before. Oh, those happy, bright lights all around you!"

"You see all that?" I was so, so hopeful.

"Yes! Now stop worrying! That bulge is not life threatening!" Charmaine was loud and clear.

She sees something so beautiful and hopeful at a time like this? But I shouldn't be surprised because she knew my mother had some good years left even when everyone else had given up on her. There really is more to this world than we know.

I drove to the clinic early in the morning and was examined right away by the doctor in charge. He assured me that the bulge was not solid or fluid filled because it had a hollow sound when he palpated it. If it had been fluid filled, the sound would not have reverberated. He managed to calm me down and urged me to keep in touch with any other concerns.

I called Charmaine later on in the day to tell her what the doctor said about my abdomen.

"Told ya," she said with a little chuckle. "There's nothing wrong with you, girl. Stop worrying."

"I'll try," I said. I felt so much better after the examination and after speaking with Charmaine.

My friend C, who is also psychic, came over the next day and put his hand close to the bulge. "There's no problem there. It's healing. I can feel a positive energy field around it. You need to calm down. You're still suffering from posttraumatic stress disorder."

"You're right about that," I said.

We sat in silence for a few minutes, and I thought about how C and Charmaine had literally walked into my life when I needed them most. They were both powerful, confident, and self-accepting people who weren't scared of the devil.

C broke the silence. "There's a story about a famous Indian guru. Crowds of sick people would gather around him, and he would simply ask them this question: 'How are you feeling?' They would all respond with the usual *monkey mind* statements, beating around the bush and discussing past traumas and future anxiety and not really answering the question. He would ask the question again: 'How are you feeling?' He tried to get them to focus on the present, to keep them in the here and now. Most of us don't live in the present. We have guilt about the past, we worry about the future, and we avoid the present moment."

"I know. Wayne Dyer talks about that on television."

"That's right. Anyway, the few people who finally managed to concentrate on the present and really perceive how they were feeling were healed right then and there. Interesting, isn't it?"

"Yes, very. I want to read Eckhart Tolle's book *The Power of Now*[9] as well."

"One of the things I'm trying to do with you is to get you to

---

[9] Eckhart Tolle, *The Power of Now* (Novato, CA: New World Publishing, 2004).

live in the present. That's all we have. Don't ruin it with negative thoughts that can't change anything anyway."

"Oh! I just remembered reading a book by Greg Anderson, *The 22 Non-Negotiable Laws of Wellness*.[10] He had metastatic lung cancer and wasn't supposed to live. He took charge of his life and noticed that people who survive serious diseases usually make a spiritual decision to live in the present and enjoy it fully."

"You'll enjoy the present when you become a whole person, accept yourself just as you are, and think of yourself as complete. It's obvious that you were expected to change yourself and deny the real you as a child. Kids who have that kind of schism in their personalities often become psychosomatic. You've got to decide what kind of person you're going to be for the rest of your life."

I stared at him while I tried to process what he was saying. I knew he was right.

We continued with a Buddhist meditation. C asked me to pretend I was holding a tiny midget in my hands, symbolic of myself as a little girl. He asked me to treat her with infinite tenderness and to tell her it was safe for her to emerge from her protective shell. I closed my eyes and focused on that image for a long time. It felt so good! I sent waves of loving energy to that little girl—my inner child.

Then we did a special exercise that is supposed to be very helpful for talking to the inner child. I wrote a question addressing the little girl with my right hand. Then I imagined what her answer would be and wrote it with my left hand. That was very awkward because I'm right-handed, but it was fun. I asked her, "Can you hear me?"

She answered, "I sure can!"

I asked her how old she was.

---

[10] Greg Anderson, *The 22 Non-Negotiable Laws of Wellness* (New York: HarperCollins, 1995).

She replied, "I'm five years old!"

I asked her how she was feeling.

"Feeling good!" Eventually she said, "Thanks for being a friend!"

C also told me it was extremely important to write letters to my late parents and to tell them exactly how I felt about everything that had happened. I did that after he left and found it to be very therapeutic. I showed the letters to him the next time he came, and he told me to keep writing them. The goal was to disarm those negative memories so they would no longer interfere with my true self.

One day he stopped short beside my dining room table. He shivered and wouldn't talk for a few minutes. "That was your father," he whispered. "I got the sense that he used to think life was just a meaningless collection of molecules. I think he's found peace and meaning now, though." I was stunned because C had never met my dad, and I had not told C about how Dad found God and peace before the end.

"That's amazing. Charmaine, my other psychic friend, says she's also seen him on the other side and that he's much happier now."

After these special inner child exercises, I began to treat myself with utmost tenderness. I would stroke my head at bedtime, as if I were my own mother, and say, "It's okay. You're going to be fine. You're such a cute little kid. Sweet dreams, kiddo."

It took me a few days to realize that I found myself talking like that to the trees, the leaves, the deer crossing the road, the bald eagles, the cats and dogs scurrying to get away from my car, the little kids in the playground close to my house, and strangers in the street. I felt more and more connected to everything that was alive, as if I were an integral part of every living thing. I looked up at a tall, dark tree that used to look forbidding and thought, *I'm part of you. I learned in chemistry class that atoms spread out almost into infinity.*

That means everything is connected no matter which way you look at it. Now I fully understand what the sages mean when they say that all our problems are caused by the illusion of self or ego as separate from other beings. It also occurred to me that psychic people may just have the rare gift of being able to perceive this connection more intensely than most of us. I was becoming a much happier person, and my fears were diminishing. I no longer felt alone.

C discussed life after death with me and suggested I look at the website of Dr. Perriakos, a physicist who had done experiments on the soul or spirit. He had scientifically measured two kinds of energy that leave a dying body: a universal and a personal energy. Several scientists concur with this research, and many psychics claim to feel similar energies. And it's common knowledge that many people who have had near-death experiences speak of flying toward a beautiful, brilliant light. All this makes me think of the famous biblical phrase: "Death, where is thy sting?"

Chapter 19

Third Chemo

I drove to N's place early one morning in the third week of November, left the car in her driveway, and got into her van for a ride to the cancer clinic, which was on her way to work. I wasn't nearly as restless during the third round of chemo, and the dreaded nausea never materialized. She picked me up in the early afternoon and took me back to her home, where I had an invigorating nap. I joined the Baha'i study group at 6:00.

The beautiful architect's daughter gave me a list of healthy superfoods to eat and a list of harmful cosmetics and other substances; a cancer nutrition expert had compiled those lists for her mother when the family was still desperately trying to save her life. Some people think one should avoid acidic foods because cancer is supposed to thrive in an acidic environment. I had already read a book about the benefits of alkaline foods. Many cosmetics contain carcinogenic chemicals, and many foods that look perfectly innocent, such as black pepper, can contain carcinogens. Overheated cooking oils become carcinogenic. The daughter told me she only wore special cosmetics that were totally natural and did not contain any petroleum-based substances. I was grateful that she bothered to print out the lists.

Everyone was eager to hear about my progress, and I was overwhelmed to hear that the whole group had been praying for me ever since they met me! The Baha'i religion, which originated in Iran in the 1800s, is a truly beautiful and peaceful religion. Most of the study group members were Iranian, and they were among the kindest, gentlest people I've ever met. Many of them had to flee from their homeland because of extreme persecution. My heart reached out to them, and I felt strongly connected to them. Apparently some of the Baha'i members had been sent to Siberia, like some of the members of my mother's family.

After spending the night at N's house, I drove back home and was amazed that I didn't feel at all dizzy or tired on the way back or for the rest of the day. I didn't even need any painkillers and had lots of energy to tackle chores around the house and go for a long walk. My bowels were working almost normally, even though the abdominal swelling was still there. My intestines became sluggish after the second round of chemo, but they normalized after the third round of chemo. I was very grateful for that because ovarian cancer can cause bowel blockages, and one can become paranoid about indigestion.

C came over a few days later and wasn't surprised to hear that I didn't need Tylenol this time. Then he came up with a fantastic insight that eased some of my pain. After reading some of the letters I wrote to my late parents, he came to the conclusion that my mother drank more than ever after my dad died because she was afraid I would take off with a man and abandon her. She figured that if she kept herself totally dependent and helpless, I wouldn't leave her. To my amazement, I suddenly forgave her completely. Medical research tells us that harboring resentment and anger only harms you.[11] One has to learn to forgive and thereby earn freedom from harmful negative emotions that only weaken one's immune system. It felt fantastic, as if the weight of the world had been lifted from my shoulders. My anger was displaced by a tender pity.

C added that when you forgive everyone else, you can forgive yourself for being unkind to yourself. *True healing can only occur when you're kind to yourself.* I was reminded of literature that advises us to send loving-kindness to the parts of our bodies that need healing. The attitude of "fighting" a disease is counterproductive. Fighting involves negativity, and that can only bring harm. Even if one's days are numbered, it's easier to pass to the other side while feeling *nothing but love*. I made a big step forward in my spiritual development on that day.

Now I fully understood and internalized the Buddhist saying, "No self, no problem." I was wiser and more profound than ever before, in spite of the fact that C said it's often very difficult for people over fifty to change in a big way.

I read books written by doctors about how best to deal with cancer. One of the most useful was Dr. Andrew Weil's *Spontaneous Healing*.[12] He recommends meditation, guided imagery, therapeutic touch, Reiki, regular exercise, organic foods, lots of fruits and vegetables, salmon, sardines, support groups, and faith in a higher power. The cancer patient will have to make changes on all levels: physical, mental/emotional, and spiritual. He noticed that the successful patients he knew were not the same people they were at the onset of the illness. Many of them made significant changes in their lives, including changes in their relationships, jobs, places of residence, diet, habits, and other things. Illness can be a gift that

---

[11] Frank Minirth and Paul Meier, *Happiness Is a Choice* (Grand Rapids, MI: Baker Books, 2007).
[12] Andrew Weil, *Spontaneous Healing* (New York: Random House, 1995).

stimulates personal growth and development, and that was certainly true in my case.

The BC Cancer Foundation says one should eat small portions of food and try to lose weight to avoid getting cancer. Worldwide studies show a correlation between obesity and cancer.[13] Animal fat and preserved meats, such as sausages and bacon, should be avoided completely because many contain carcinogenic nitrites. There is evidence that red meat and processed meat are a cause of colorectal cancer, and this information was recently published in the Cancer Prevention Research journal. Too much alcohol is also associated with cancer. Cases of heart disease and cancer are lower in countries that use only olive oil for cooking. If you've already had cancer, following these guidelines can help prevent a relapse.

More recent news, which I suspected long ago, is that not getting enough sleep makes your immune system vulnerable to attack and less able to fight off potentially cancerous cells.[14] Night shift workers are especially vulnerable to cancer. One should try everything possible to get a good night's sleep. If you think you need a new mattress, get one. Try taking a warm bath before bed and learning to relax completely. Herbal muscle relaxants may help, as may focusing on breathing to drown out busy thoughts.

By the time the third round of chemo hurdle was over, I was a new woman. I really meant it with a passion when I told myself, "I love you," and I could stand in front of the mirror at any time of the day or night and say it. I took very good care of myself and had become my own best friend.

---

[13] *Cancer Prevention Research,* July 2010. 3:852.
[14] "Lack of Sleep Affects Body's Immune System." *Healthbeat,* abc7 News, WLS-TV Chicago, July 2, 2012.

Chapter 20

Radiation

I went to the BC Cancer Agency in Vancouver early in December to see the oncology team for postchemo assessment and to prepare for the radiation treatments. Dr. O gave me a thorough pelvic exam and found no evidence of tumor recurrence. I also was pleasantly surprised to hear that he considered me to be a poster girl for chemo. He was amazed that, in his words, "something in my body" eliminated the chemicals quickly. He had been studying the results of the lab tests as I was undergoing chemo and was pleased to see that my blood consistently recovered from the assault on my system. He showed me some of the results and said that my tumor was a "class-two, well-behaved cyst" and that I had an "80 to 82 percent chance of living another fifteen years." I had mixed feelings about that. It was good to hear I wasn't expected to pass away in just a few years, but the fifteen-year limit made me squirm. *Would my time really be up after fifteen years?*

He asked me about my sex life, and it reminded me of a recent worldwide study I had read in the health section of the CBC Internet news.[15] According to the study, single people who have never been married and don't have kids or other family support have smaller chances of surviving major illnesses. Similar recent studies seem to agree with this, indicating that married people have higher survival rates from life-threatening diseases. I thought to myself, *Great. After all this effort, that's what I have to look forward to—a lower chance of surviving to really enjoy life? Not fair at all.* On the other hand, these studies prove how important love really is and how it can make all the difference between life and death no matter how many hospital visits one makes. Well, I now have a heart big enough to love the whole world, whether it loves me back or not. That love will sustain me for the rest of my life. If I was a poster girl for chemo, maybe I'll be a poster girl for radiation. I can't give up now. I'll ignore the depressing research on single people. I know single people who have lived well into their nineties.

A nurse guided me to the CT scan area, and I was given some reading material about radiation treatments and how to prepare for them. After I undressed, a technician helped me onto a stretcher beside a computerized scanner. She marked my abdomen with little black dots that would be used to guide the radiation beams when I returned in a week to begin the treatment. I was to buy a high-quality moisturizer so I would be prepared for skin irritation. My first treatment was to be on December 15—the anniversary of the day my mother passed away.

I looked at the lovely Christmas trees and other decorations in the area when the marking session was over. *Merry Christmas to you, kid. If the radiation will help to save your life, that will be the best present of all. You've got too much living to do.*

N, my Baha'i friend, wanted me to stay in her Vancouver apartment for the first month of the radiation. I packed my car

---

15 "Being in Love is Good for the Heart." www.cbn.com/cbnnews/healthscience/2012/February.

with some clothes and books, picked up the keys, took the ferry, and drove to the downtown apartment. It was a loft apartment way up in a high-rise close to the Granville Street Bridge. It had a partial view of the North Shore Mountains and Burrard Inlet and was close to the trendy Yaletown shops and restaurants.

I drove myself to my treatments, which lasted about fifteen to twenty minutes each, and then I was free to enjoy the city. I walked in the downtown area frequently and was pleased to be able to do that without getting too tired. I bought a juicer and used it every day because I had heard that juices are easily absorbed by the digestive system and that the nutrients get into the system quickly. I tried all sorts of fruit and vegetable combinations and had fun experimenting with that. A good old friend from my student days at UBC was very supportive, picking me up at the cancer agency one day and taking me for lunch and for a beautiful, long walk in the university area.

The radiation units opened early in the morning and operated late into the evening. There were many men and women of all ages waiting for treatments. We all had storage bags for our treatment gowns, and we would change into them in cubicles and then wait for the friendly technicians to call us. I would lie down on a table under a big, bulb-like device that would rotate around my body, and there was a zapping noise that lasted only a few seconds. I closed my eyes and tried to relax completely. I had to be lined up so that my black dot markers were in place, and I had to be careful not to breathe heavily while the machine was emitting radiation. *Energy of healing light, come into my body and make sure there are no more cancer cells anywhere.*

The treatments were done on Monday through Friday, and I would visit the agency's lab once a week so the radiation oncologist could check my immune system. If my white cell count would go down too low, I would be in danger of a serious infection. Sometimes I would drive to the ferry terminal and go back home for the weekend, especially if the Monday treatment was later in the afternoon or in the evening. Once, close to Christmas, I decided to take the bus to the terminal. The bus could not make it down the steep hill into town, so I had to walk in the snow with regular street shoes all the way to the ferry. I had just been warned that my white cell count was dangerously low. I was wearing a very warm coat, but my shoes were not adequate, and my feet were freezing. I was amazed that I didn't catch a cold.

After Christmas, I developed nausea during the treatments. One of the doctors suggested I buy Gravol because she didn't think it would be a good idea to overload my body with prescription drugs. I chewed on the tablets frequently and occasionally threw up. When my regular oncologist came back from holidays, he prescribed stronger antinausea medication, and that helped a lot.

In the middle of January, with only two weeks of radiation left, I moved into the basement suite of some doctor friends. They were very kind, often asking me upstairs for dinner and frequently checking up on my progress. The three family cats provided me with an endless source of amusement. I began to have rectal bleeding—one of the symptoms of treatment—and used a prescription ointment to treat it. I also had to take a cab to the clinic during the last week because my nausea made it impossible to drive. The volunteer drivers stopped at 5:00, and many of my treatments were late in the evening. The drugs were not always very effective. Dr. R, my radiation oncologist, also confessed that at one point he had been worried I would not be able to finish the treatments because of a compromised immune system.

I was thrilled to get back home in February and enjoyed my garden more than ever before. The plants never looked so good or so welcoming! I grinned at the eagles and herons as they flew over my house, my hair started growing back little by little, and I pampered myself with facials and pedicures.

I had an abdominal CT scan and then went back to Vancouver for a follow up in March. Dr. O was pleased with the results. He wished me a long life and told me I could travel anywhere I wanted. I was happy that he liked my short hair because I planned to keep it that way. Dr. R was as friendly and as humorous as usual and told me not to worry too much about follow-ups. I was referred back to Dr. A in Nanaimo.

I felt so free, and I wanted to go everywhere at once. I had never been to the Far East, so I went to Japan with a Japanese friend and stayed in her family's house in Chigasaki, which is close to Tokyo. We saw the great Buddha at Kamakura, explored Yokohama, went to the foothills of Mt. Fuji with her friends, and walked to the beach and to the island of Enoshima. We ate exotic foods and took the *Shinkansen,* or high-speed bullet train, to Kyoto and Nara. I was particularly inspired by the Buddhist temples because C had introduced me to Buddhist teachings during my chemo treatments. The plane trips did not tire me too much, and I had plenty of energy for sightseeing. That was a good sign.

I went to New Mexico with a good friend in October, and I loved Santa Fe. When I returned, I had a CT scan at the hospital and was immensely relieved to hear that there was no sign of a relapse. That gave me the confidence to plan a trip to Europe with a group of friends for the first time in thirteen years.

In April 2007, we flew to Amsterdam and took a river boat from Amsterdam to Budapest, going on the Rhine, Main, and Danube Rivers. After the cruise, I flew by myself to Copenhagen, then Oslo, and then Stockholm. I took the ferry to Tallinn to see my cousins in Estonia and to finally get a feeling of closure about my mom.

One cousin took me to see the grave of my mom's sister. In broken English, he told me that my aunt had died of an abdominal cancer in an organ that only females have. Cancer and heart disease ran in the family, and I realized there might have been a genetic component to my own abdominal cancer.

On another day, he drove his mother and me to another cemetery to see the grave of his sister, who was my only female cousin. The midafternoon sun warmed my back as I watched my cousin's mother kneel beside the grave and place a little pot of delicate flowers in front of the shiny black headstone.

"Can you hear me? Listen to me!" she said, her voice shrill with grief even though my cousin had passed away seven years before.

I stared at the inscribed dates on the stone and felt a hot tear roll down my cheek. My cousin was barely forty-three when she succumbed to a very aggressive double breast cancer. Many young Estonians were dying of cancer around that time because the Soviets had poisoned the environment with nuclear waste. Even though the new democratic government was working hard to make the environment safer, the Soviet legacy was still oppressive.

"See lovely flowers?" my cousin's mother asked. I was surprised to hear her speak English because I knew she really didn't know the language. She seemed to be in a trance and sounded as if she was truly expecting an answer.

I thought back to the June day in 1991 when I first met my cousin at her parents' country home close to Tallinn. My mom, who hadn't been back home for forty-seven years because of the cold war, was elated to be having supper with her beloved brother (my cousin's father) and the rest of his family, and I was delighted to be meeting everyone for the first time. My cousin's baby boy was asleep in a crib close to the dining room.

After dinner, my cousin took me upstairs to her small bedroom. I sat down on her woven bedspread and admired the pretty pea green and yellow pattern. I traced some of the designs with my finger.

"I made it," she said with a slight smile. "Sorry, my English not so good."

"But you're doing very well. I'm sorry I don't know Estonian," I said.

She showed me other cute handicrafts, including a small stuffed pig with a comical face, and told me how much she enjoyed making them. Then she produced a stack of black-and-white pictures. "We are training here," she said as she showed me a picture of her with several friends, all of them wearing helmets and paddling on a river raft.

"Wow, you all look so athletic," I said.

"Yes, we are training on Estonian river to be ready to go to Lake Baikal."

I was impressed. She and her fearless friends were aiming to go whitewater rafting deep within the Soviet Union. She was tall and sinewy and had thick, dark hair that framed her sculptured features.

"You know, I wanted to write to you all these years, but Mom and I were scared of the KGB. We had heard too many horror stories about innocent people being sent back to Siberia for having contact with the West," I said, speaking slowly. I looked deep into her eyes, trying to make her understand. I'm not sure if she did or not.

Then she showed me another picture of her group sitting around a campfire. "That is my son's father," she said as she pointed at a stocky blond man.

"Oh. Where is he now?" He wasn't downstairs with the rest of the family.

"I don't know. We are not married." She looked dejected and forlorn.

"Does he visit you and your son?" I asked hopefully.

"No." She shook her head.

I gasped.

"He told me he was not married, and I fell in love with him." There was a big lump in her throat. "I thought he want to marry me when I was pregnant. Then he said he was already married."

"Oh, how awful. He lied to you." I touched her hand.

Mom and I left Estonia just before the coup against Gorbachev and went back in August 1994, when the country was already independent. When we arrived at Mom's brother's house one afternoon, my cousin's son was in the front garden laughing and chasing his friends with the fury of a dust devil. My cousin was laughing like a child too as she watched him leap and lurch all over the place.

After supper, my cousin and I strolled around the garden. "Would you like to see the school where I teach? I could take you there tomorrow," she said. She looked smart in her blue jeans and burgundy sweater.

"I'd love to," I said without hesitation.

She arrived at my downtown Tallinn hotel the next morning, and we took a bus that went past a building that looked like an academic institution. "That is where I became a teacher," she said.

"Oh, good for you," I said.

She was silent for a couple of minutes. "I am sad because I did not get into Tartu University. That is where the best students go. I am not smart enough."

I knew that Tartu was one of the oldest and best universities in northern Europe, but it wasn't the only place to study. "But you are a teacher," I said in a flattering tone.

"Yes, but I don't make enough money to look after my son. I may have to learn computers to make more money." She gave a heavy sigh.

We arrived at the elementary school, which was in a wooded area. It had three floors, and there were a few kids playing under the trees. "School will start again soon. I miss the children." She used her key to open a side door, and we walked up a couple of flights of stairs to her classroom.

"What grade do you teach?" I asked her.

"Grade two," she said happily.

"Oh look, there's your name over the door," I said as I pointed to the sign.

We walked around the room, which had a nice view of the yard, and admired some brown paper drawings that were in a neat pile on a supply table. "The school does not have enough money, so I bring things from home. I like to keep the children busy," she said in a warm tone.

We looked around a little more before going back down the stairs and out to the yard. "Maybe they will raise teacher salaries soon," I said. "After all, the government is different now."

My cousin gave a hopeless shrug. "Maybe."

We spent several hours in the endlessly fascinating medieval town, walking in and out of museums, churches, arts and crafts shops, and coffee shops. I felt so close to her that I wished I were a fairy godmother with enough magical powers to make her life happier.

"See lovely flowers?" My cousin's mother repeated her question and jolted me back into the present afternoon at my cousin's grave.

Another hot tear rolled down my cheek. *It's such a pity that you had to leave us too soon. I would have enjoyed telling you all about my cancer journey and how I learned to love and accept myself. I might have been able to help you do the same for yourself.*

Chapter 21

Through the Fire

One of my friends convinced me to join her Tuesday-evening ladies' Bible study class at her church, which is only a few blocks away from my house. I had not studied the Bible seriously since I was in Sunday school, but I'm always receptive to spiritual growth in any form, so I agreed to go. My first class was eleven days after my October 5 abdominal CT scan, and I was quite anxious because I had not heard anything about the results, which are usually available within two or three days. I was beginning to think they had to send the results to Vancouver for further analysis. I was especially agitated because Dr. A had told me that most of relapses happened within the first two years after the diagnosis of my particular type of ovarian cancer. *Would I still be cancer free?*

We watched a video made by Beth Moore, a Bible scholar, about the third chapter of Daniel, in which Shadrach, Meshach, and Abednego were delivered *through the fire* with a mysterious fourth man at their side. King Nebuchadnezzar had ordered the three men to be thrown into his fiery furnace because they would not worship him. He was stunned to see that they survived it without a scratch or a burn and that the fourth man looked like a son of the gods.

Beth explained that we encounter fires in our own lives. Some people suffer with cancer; that is just one example of a fiery trial. She went on to explain that sometimes God delivers us *from* the fire (we don't have to go through the trial), sometimes God delivers us *through* the fire (we go through, but we come out of it alive), and sometimes He delivers us *by* the fire (we die and go into His arms). Jesus is the fourth man, and He helps us through it all. No matter what happens, a fire that can never be extinguished is lit in someone's heart. These are gripping images, and one doesn't have to be religious in any way to feel their power and relevance.

We discussed the video as we sat at a large, round table and then shared our private concerns so we could all pray for each other. When my turn came to share, I told the group how worried I was about my CT scan results. Of course, I had to briefly summarize my experience with cancer so they would know what to pray for. When I finished, one lady exclaimed, "You've been through the fire!" I stared at her and nodded slowly.

My friend prayed out loud, asking God to help each woman in the group with her problems. She asked Him to give me the results of the scan soon so I would be at peace and stop worrying. It was such a lovely, sweet feeling to connect with everyone in such a beautiful, empathic way. Most of these ladies were total strangers until that evening, and they took turns praying out loud for each other.

On the way home it suddenly occurred to me that I should write a short booklet about my experience with ovarian cancer, publish it myself, sell it as a fundraiser, and give all the proceeds for research that would focus on finding a test for early detection so fewer and fewer women would have to actually go through the fire. We've all heard the famous phrase, "The Lord works in mysterious ways." I had often wondered if the Creator had a special plan for me, and this project certainly seemed to be part of it.

The booklets were distributed for awareness and for fundraising, and many people who read the booklet sent checks to Dr. Brad Nelson's ovarian cancer research lab at the Cancer Agency in Victoria. Some people also told me that reading the booklet gave them more courage to face all the problems in their lives.

I love and accept myself so fully now that I want to share this feeling with everyone.

Chapter 22

An Attitude of Gratitude

One of the books that has greatly improved and enriched my life is *Learn to Be an Optimist: A Practical Guide to Achieving Happiness* by Lucy MacDonald.[16] I found a copy in a used bookstore about two years after my treatments were finished.

One chapter discusses keeping an optimism journal. This kind of journal can have all kinds of applications, such as using it to list the things for which you should be grateful, to face your fears, or to track your level of happiness over time. The author informs us that by exploring your reaction to the major and minor events in your life, you can reach a better understanding of how you think—a first step toward increasing your optimism. When I heard Dr. Daniel Amen speak on public television about how great it is for your brain to actually write down the things you can be grateful for instead of just thinking about them, I realized that a *gratitude* journal would become a new daily habit for me.

---

[16] Lucy MacDonald, *Learn to Be an Optimist* (San Francisco, CA: Chronicle Books, 2004).

We've heard this many times before, but it really is useful to count our blessings. Ms. MacDonald suggests asking yourself, "What do I have to be grateful for?" You can start with absolutely anything that occurs to you. Perhaps you could start with the basics, like having a roof over your head, food to eat, family, and friends, and then list recent positive events, such as goals you have achieved or times when someone has been kind to you. If necessary, walk around your home and use all five of your senses to appreciate it. You might be grateful for beautiful music, your pets, a delicious meal, the lovely scent of soap, or the feel of a new towel against your skin. At the end of the day, write down your list of blessings, big and small, and reflect upon them.

Following are a few of my gratitude journal entries.

March 15, 2008
I'm very grateful that my good friend accompanied me to Victoria! It's always uplifting and inspiring to go there, and it was wonderful to see so many gorgeous blooming trees. I love the delicate pink ornamental cherry blossoms that always appear earlier down there than in my midisland area. It's like leaving winter behind and driving right into spring.

The pool at the hotel was very relaxing, and the staff members were all friendly. We loved our bean and lentil soup at the health food restaurant close to the hotel, and the rooftop restaurant had terrific appetizers in the evening. Downtown Victoria is beautiful from any angle, but seeing the city lights from above was a special treat. It was a good way to end the day after spending a couple of hours at the hospital seminar room listening to Dr. Rob Rutledge, the radiation oncologist, and Dr. Tim Walker, the psychologist.

Even though my treatments finished early in 2006, I have a few years to go before I reach the five-years-cancer-free mark, and I want to do everything it takes to stay healthy so I don't have a relapse. I learned a lot at the seminar—things that are useful for *everyone,* not just cancer patients and survivors.

Dr. Rob and Dr. Tim told us how important it is to slow ourselves down and take care of ourselves. We sometimes get so busy that we forget to calm down, but the deeper levels of wisdom appear when you *slow down.*

Pray to accept whatever arises, and *love yourself.*

Exercise is the most important thing you can do to get well. It strengthens you and releases endorphins, or happy hormones, that de-stress you.

Stick to a low-fat diet. Change the "blood soup" around the cancer cells, because it's the soup of chemicals around them that caused them to mutate to begin with. Create "happy genetics."

Listen to your body. When do you feel good? Do what makes you feel good, and be *grateful* to your body. We're all *walking miracles.*

Try to sleep well and relax. Chi Gong exercises slow down the heartbeat and the "chatting mind." The brain changes no matter how old you are, so influence your brain in a positive way. If you start the day in a relaxing way, it's good for you and percolates through you all day.

Create time and space for things you like to do, and say no to things you don't like. Cut out nonessentials, seek bliss, and have good hobbies.

Meditate. Concentrate on your breath to forget busy thoughts. Meditate to be with the divine.

We have to face our fears, and there is nothing to fear but fear itself.

We must integrate our spirits, minds, and physical bodies.

Dr. Rob and Dr. Tim are so kind and caring!

It was a pleasure to visit their website: www.robrutledge.ca.

The doctors also said that the power of the cancer journey is: "How can I love?" I agree with that, and I think I have tried hard to reach out and love others by writing the *Through the Fire* booklet. I'm also planning to volunteer at the Canadian Cancer Society soon and help with raising funds for pediatric cancer research and for Camp Goodtimes, an amusement park for kids with cancer. I'll be helping to coordinate the midisland Tour de Rock, in which police officers ride their bikes all around Vancouver Island. They're incredibly dedicated, and they train for months for the kids. It brings the community together in very a warm and loving way.

As much as I love Victoria, I love the midisland area just as much. I really enjoyed visiting wildlife recovery centers and farms today. I saw an adorable barred owl and an eagle that will stay at the recovery center. I also bought some chocolate sauce at the farm gift store and got a kick out of the calves and the lamb. Another friend took me to a petting zoo, and we saw a Shetland pony, two black-and-white calves, a Sicilian donkey, a baby white sheep, newborn goats, lots of rabbits and chickens, and some bronze turkeys. We laughed when the Muscovy duck hissed at us. All the animals were too cute for words. It felt so good to be with the animals today. They live in the present, and they're so playful that they can lift your spirit. I must visit them more often!

October 1, 2008

I had a fabulous day! My gynecologist thinks I'm already cured, even though it's only been three years since my chemo started. He told me that when my type of ovarian cancer recurs, it's usually within the first two years. And he said my abdominal MRI was perfect and "couldn't be better." I am so grateful to modern medicine and to my dedicated doctors.

I also think I've helped myself a lot by *living more in the moment* and travelling to so many fabulous places on my bucket list, like Florence and Venice. My friend and I had a terrific time there and met so many interesting people on the cruise from Southampton to

Venice. Dubrovnik was also fantastic, and it was so heartwarming to see it free from oppression.

May 9, 2009

A friend and I took the twenty-minute ferry ride from Nanaimo to Gabriola Island and had a great time. We went straight to the Haven resort, a place of spiritual healing established by two medical doctors. It has a lovely setting right by the ocean, and we had green ginger tea in the little restaurant. We walked around and talked about how nice it would be to come back, stay for a healing weekend, and go to spiritual growth workshops. Some of my other friends go there regularly and love it.

Then we went to the Folklife village with the old-fashioned boardwalks around the stores and had delicious veggie sandwiches while admiring stained glass art in the gift shop. We were amazed at the beauty of the marina in Silva Bay, and the hotel owner showed us one of the comfortable kitchenette suites so we would be inspired to go back. Gabriola is a warm, cozy island with friendly, happy people. I look forward to visiting again.

May 21–22, 2009

The drive over the mountains to the west coast of Vancouver Island was spectacular! I've never seen the mountains look so clear and imposing, so majestic and huge. It was a mystical and powerful experience that made me realize how small my problems really are in the grand scheme of things.

I was very surprised to see how much bigger Ucluelet is now. It has lovely new west coast–style buildings and more high-quality art galleries. We stood at the edge of the main dock, and a big brown harbor seal suddenly emerged from the ocean depths, snorted, and dove down again. It seemed to be welcoming us to Ucluelet.

We walked on the wild Pacific trail for a while and admired

the rocky islands and the waves crashing against the dark rocks beneath us.

We stayed at the Tin Wis ("calm waters") hotel in Tofino, and we loved walking on the hard, rippled sand on the beach. There's even a gourmet sushi restaurant in Tofino. It's hard to believe there are so many amenities in a place that used to be very remote.

September 2010

My gynecologist shook my hand and told me I was cancer-free for five years. I have reached the mark that all cancer patients aim and hope for, and I couldn't possibly be more grateful.

March 2011

My first trip to South America was fascinating! I loved Lima and Machu Picchu in Peru. Then I went on a cruise from Santiago to the Chilean fjords, around Cape Horn and Tierra del Fuego, and to Montevideo and Sao Paulo. I was amazed that so many people spoke English. I was very pleased that I didn't suffer too much from the high altitude in the Andes, partly because I drank lots of coca leaf tea in the hotel and took the prescription medication my doctor gave me. I had a terrific guide in Santiago—a retired engineer who showed me the mansions that were used as prisons by the Pinochet regime. I felt lucky to be alive and felt so sorry for those innocent souls who disappeared without a trace.

I really enjoyed hearing a lady Buddhist monk from Seattle speak at a local church for the Lenten lecture series. She said, "Suffering is very real, and we're here to help each other through it." How much more profound and meaningful can you get?

I feel a tender, infinite love for myself, for every other living thing, and even for the objects in my house all around me, as if every machine has a soul and wants to help make my life easier.

Someone sent me an e-mail message about an eighty-seven-year-old lady who just earned a college degree. She advises us all to always keep our dreams alive, to never stop playing, to look for the humorous, funny things every day, and to have no regrets.

I must say, I love living here and have no regrets about moving here. I have met so many warm and dedicated people who work tirelessly to make our community the best it can be.

April 16, 2011

I went to a pastor-led meditation centering prayer at a nearby church. A candle was lit for our half-hour silent prayer. After the prayer, some people confessed they were hoping to find God's purpose for them.

I was so grateful that I already knew what my main purpose was: to be a good, empathic friend to many and to help, teach, and inspire others with words and music.

April 20, 2011

Today I learned that Canada is the second-happiest country in the world! We're tied with Sweden, right behind Denmark. That is really something to be grateful for. Too many countries in our world don't seem to know what happiness is.

February 6, 2012

My doctor called to tell me that my DEXA bone density test was much better than it was two years ago. Long after my treatments were over, I found out that the chemo and radiation had damaged my spine, putting it in the osteoporotic range, but Actonel (a drug that stops the breakdown of bone) and lots of weight-bearing exercise and high-quality calcium and magnesium supplements, more calcium-rich foods, and less caffeine obviously helped me. He suggested that I stay on Actonel for another three years because one usually takes bisphosphonates for five years.

I am so grateful and happy to know that osteoporosis can be reversed and will do whatever it takes to keep my bones strong from now on. I love going to *Curves*, which has been approved by the Board of Osteoporosis Canada because its resistance training machines can strengthen bones.

February 25, 2012
I attended a wonderful emotional freedom technique (EFT) group session today!

A very empathic and accomplished young lady healer led the group, and we learned a lot about the theory and practice of this technique, which was founded by Gary Craig and based upon the energy meridians that were discovered by the Chinese thousands of years ago.

Western scientists have proven the existence of these meridians, and the tapping technique that one can perform on oneself is so effective it helps some soldiers alleviate posttraumatic stress disorder.

Even if you haven't been in a war, daily life throws all sorts of challenges at you, and if you don't get rid of negative emotions caused by toxic encounters, you waste a lot of valuable energy just licking your wounds. This is energy that could be used in happier, more fulfilling ways.

Learning to use EFT on yourself is an act of self-love and self-acceptance. In fact, you're even supposed to tell yourself, for example, "Even though I'm still angry that my boss called me stupid, *I completely love and accept myself*" while you tap on various energy points on your body.

Chapter 23

Edward and Bianca

Edward was dreaming that he was back in the war. As a commander in the British army, he was responsible for his men, but he couldn't help them now. They were surrounded by thick, pungent smoke and could hardly breathe. *What the hell? We've never been caught unprepared like this.* He coughed violently and gasped for air.

He woke up, but he wondered if he was still dreaming. His eyes were stinging, and he was sweating as if he were naked in the desert sun. *Am I back in Egypt? Or India?*

Good God, my bed is on fire! He leaped off the bed, ran to the bedroom door, flung it open, stood at the top of the stairs, and called out to his wife.

There was no answer.

He ran downstairs, grabbed the fire extinguisher, ran back upstairs, and sprayed the entire hot, stinking, smoking mattress until he smothered the blaze. Then the alarm clock went off.

"Ruddy clock—you're a bit late, aren't you?" he said to the clock as he silenced it. *I've got an important staff meeting this morning, and I don't even have time to dwell on the fact that my bed was on fire and that I could have choked to death.* He showered and dressed quickly, went downstairs to the kitchen, and poured himself a glass of orange juice. *I can get a quick breakfast in the cafeteria at work, but I'd better check the rest of the house before I leave.*

There didn't seem to be any sign of an intruder. *Bloody hell.* Then he remembered that his wife had recently suspected him of having an affair, that she had shown a propensity for extreme violence very soon after they got married twenty years before, and that she was capable of hysterical behavior. Just before Christmas a few months before, she had swallowed a fistful of sleeping pills while standing next to the phone and then called for an ambulance. Her stomach was pumped out at the hospital, and she survived beautifully with no lingering aftereffects. *She set my bed on fire. There's no point in calling the police.* He gave a long, labored sigh.

He got into his car. *The stress of managing a big downtown bank is nothing compared to living with my maniacal wife. Heck, the stress of the war was nothing compared to this.*

* * * * *

Bianca's eyes bulged as her husband tightened his grip on her throat. "*Una vida regala*, that's what you have, and it's not good enough for you!" he shouted as his face crimsoned.

How am I going to get this madman to stop? I can't even scream for help. I'm too young to die. There must be something I can do. Think, think, think, before it's too late. My nails! They're strong and sharp. She sunk her nails into his face as hard as she could, her adrenalin giving her the extraordinary power she needed to shock him into releasing her.

Hyperventilating, she ran to the front door and was out in the front yard before he could stop her. A friendly neighbor was pruning bushes just a few feet away. "Are you all right? I've never seen you so pale," she said as she walked toward Bianca.

"I … am not … very well, but … at least I am still alive," Bianca said with a weak, trembling voice between gasps for air.

"Is there anything I can do? Shall I call a doctor?" The neighbor touched Bianca's arm tenderly.

"I think I am going to have to move out and call a lawyer," Bianca said with a steadier voice.

"Oh, it must be that nasty husband of yours. I've heard him shouting at you before."

Bianca nodded.

"If he comes out here, I'll jab him with these," the neighbor said as she waved the shears back and forth.

Bianca managed a little giggle even though she was still trembling.

"Why don't you come inside for a while, and I'll make tea? It'll calm you down and give you a chance to plan your next move." She sounded as if she were Bianca's older sister.

"Thank you, thank you," Bianca said. "And may I use your phone?"

"Of course," her neighbor said as she led her up the stairs to the front door.

Bianca sat at the kitchen table while her neighbor put the kettle on, and her breathing rate stabilized as she glanced out the window. She saw several mature cherry, pear, and apple trees, and her neighbor's big calico cat was leaping around the backyard like a playful kitten. It was such a calming, delightful sight that she forgot, for an instant, that she had been fighting for her life just a few minutes before and was still scared that her husband would rush over and attack her.

Tea was served, and after a few sips, Bianca asked if she could use the phone so she could tell her best friend about the latest crisis in her life.

"Go ahead, and take as long as you want." Her neighbor pointed to the phone, which was sitting on the kitchen counter.

Bianca was terribly nervous. *Please, please be home and answer the phone.*

After about ten rings, her friend answered. She had been out in the garden, and her sixth sense told her she needed to answer it. "Okay, that's it. I'm coming over to pick you up. Stay at your neighbor's place until I get there, and then we'll go together to your house so you can quickly pick up what you need most. Then you're moving in with us, and I'll help you get a lawyer." She spoke with great determination and confidence, giving Bianca hope that her life could be salvaged.

After Bianca's neighbor heard the whole story, she offered to come with them to help Bianca gather her belongings. "And if we have to break in, in case he's gone out and locked the doors, I've got the tools to do it." She gave a conspiratorial and confident smile that warmed Bianca's heart and mollified her fears.

Soon after Bianca moved in with her best friend, she met Edward at a dinner party, and their mutual attraction was so strong they hardly noticed what they were eating. There were at least twenty other guests at the party, so they didn't feel guilty about receding into the private little sunroom after dinner and telling each other the stories of their lives.

"My word, you are so striking and exotic. What part of Spain are you from?" Edward's gaze was steady and intense.

"I am a *Madrileña*," Bianca said in a singsong tone of voice. "I had to leave *España* because of the civil war. We went to France first and then to Mexico. That is where I married my crazy husband—the one who tried to strangle me. He teaches languages at the university, and he gave many parties for his professor friends. He expected me to mark student papers, to cook gourmet meals for his friends, and do all the housework, the sewing, and the gardening. No matter what I did, it wasn't good enough, and he and his friends would tell me, 'You are beautiful, yes, but you are not educated.' They ate my food and loved it, but they made me feel stupid. My husband was ashamed of me also because I love to laugh and dance flamenco and play castanets and wear bright red dresses. He would often tell me to change clothes and stop laughing so much. 'You are too exuberant,' he would say. 'You must learn to control yourself.' How can I change my character now? And why should I change for a man who is never happy anyway? *Ay caramba.*" She curled her lip.

Edward shook his head in a gesture of sympathy and held her hand tenderly. "Good Lord, you've been through hell, but it doesn't show. You are so radiant I can't … I can't stop staring at you. I hope that doesn't make you uncomfortable." His voice was soft and soothing.

"No, no." Bianca laughed like a little girl, making Edward grin like a sly schoolboy.

Then he told her about his violent and hysterical wife and was delighted when Bianca exploded with infectious laughter. He found himself laughing heartily about waking up on a burning mattress and couldn't believe it. *This is some woman. She's so lovely and feminine, and she makes me laugh like never before. She may look fragile, but she's incredibly resilient. Wow.*

Bianca thought, *Poor Eduardo. He's such a wonderful man, and he's been through as much hell as I have, wandering all around the world and getting stuck with crazy people. And he has such good manners and looks like a real gentleman. Where has he been all my life?*

They left the party together and didn't give a fig about what the hosts or the other guests thought about that. Edward moved out of his house and into an apartment so he could seriously court Bianca, and they went out frequently and enjoyed themselves so much they felt whole again. It was as if they each had magic wands capable of healing the other's fractured soul. And Bianca's friend found a lawyer who helped her get a fair divorce.

Edward wasn't so lucky; his wife didn't want to give him a divorce, hired a detective, and stalked him and Bianca relentlessly. One evening Edward's wife appeared in a restaurant parking lot as they got out of the car, took several pictures of them, screamed at Bianca, and called her a prostitute. On another evening, she and her detective accosted Edward as he tried to enter his apartment building.

Bianca noticed her ex-husband appearing here and there as well, as if he had also hired a detective to track her and Edward. "Can you believe this?" Bianca whispered one evening in a restaurant as she tilted her head toward the door. "*Arriva el tormentor.* He is watching us with his tiny blue eyes."

Edward and Bianca screamed with laughter, and when they recovered, they decided to go to Mexico and stay with Bianca's family. That way they could arrange for Edward's divorce and then get married.

They went on a world cruise for their honeymoon and lived happily ever after.

I met Bianca and Edward when I was very young. They were close family friends, and their lighthearted humor and resilience in the face of disaster never ceased to amaze me. They always came out on top and treated me as if I were a cherished niece. They loved and accepted me fully, and whenever something went wrong in my life, they made me laugh so hard I nearly fell off my chair. They didn't let anyone get them down for long, and they encouraged me to be the same way.

They were lucky they found each other, and I was lucky to have met them. Even though Edward passed away years ago and Bianca moved far away to live with her nephew because she can't look after herself anymore, their spirits are still with me and they still inspire me. We should all have people like that in our lives—people who love us just the way we are and can laugh, dance, and sing while everyone else is crying.

Chapter 24

Corazon

Ted craned his neck to gaze at the mysterious, monumental mountains as the short train snaked its way through the valley toward Machu Picchu in the early afternoon. He was mesmerized by the otherworldly splendor of the dramatic, misty green landscape and didn't want to miss anything. The soft Peruvian folk music that streamed out of the train's speakers was so cheerful that his soul wanted to dance, but the primitive wind instruments also spoke of an ancient, profound wisdom that seemed to know the secrets of life and death.

He was only forty, but he owned several luxury car dealerships and was exceedingly wealthy. His wife had just divorced him because she claimed he was a workaholic who didn't have time for her. In spite of the divorce, he was still rich because there were no kids to support. Even though he was very rich, he was very lonely and hoping that a trip to a place as exotic as Machu Picchu would help him feel alive again.

He couldn't concentrate too much on his loneliness because the train was bursting with excited tourists from all over the world. A blond, athletic-looking, middle-aged Brit was standing in the aisle a few steps ahead, talking to a group of Germans about his extensive travels all over South America; a large group of Chinese people from Taiwan were listening to their Chinese Brazilian tour guide; and there were several Americans, Canadians, and other Europeans.

The train suddenly lurched, slowed down, and stopped. Some fit people got up, picked up their bulky backpacks, and headed toward the doors. They were ambitious enough to hike the Inca trail up to Machu Picchu, so they crossed over the tracks and headed to the trail, which Ted could clearly see from his window. *I should be hiking up that trail, but I have to watch my heart. Those damn palpitations. All I need now is to collapse on the trail. We're so far away from any good hospitals. I hope the high-altitude pills my doctor gave me before I left home will continue to work. Heck, I'd have to be taken back to Cusco and then on to Lima, and I doubt that these backward people would be able to save me. Maybe I should have stayed home in Florida. But I need a break.* Ted's thoughts were a jumble of negatives, and he had to force himself to squash them and come back to the gift of the exotic present.

Ted was relieved when the train shuddered and moved forward because he could forget about his heart and be distracted by the anticipation of reaching the ruins. He kept his face glued to the window for the next ten minutes.

"*Señor?* You like coffee?" a young lady attendant asked with a warm, soft voice.

Ted turned his head to look at her and drew in a sudden sharp breath. She was as lovely and as mysterious as the landscape; it was as if she had just sprung out of the warm Peruvian earth.

"*Señor?*" Her voice was tentative, but her smoldering eyes betrayed a passionate, strong-willed character and a heart as big as the mountains.

Ted looked at the name plate pinned on the left side of her tailored white blouse. *Corazon* was on top of *Peru Rail*. When he recovered from his gasp, Ted said, "Yes, I'll have some coffee, thank you."

Corazon nodded. "*Con leche, señor?*" She gave him a maternally sweet smile.

"*Non, negro.* Just black, thank you." Ted couldn't stop staring at her.

"Ah, *solo?*" She raised her eyebrows.

"Si, solo," Ted whispered.

Corazon gave him a small cup of coffee, and when he touched her slender fingers during the transfer from one hand to another, he trembled a little.

"You okay, señor?" Corazon asked, looking concerned.

"Yes, I'm okay. Thank you." Ted cleared his throat and paused before he could continue. "Will you be coming with us to Machu Picchu, or will you go back to Cusco after we arrive?"

"Oh, I have day off after this, and I stay with cousins in village for the night." She was radiant.

"Please come with me and be my tour guide today. Please. I'll pay you well," Ted begged.

A hint of suspicion passed over Corazon's eyes.

"Please come with me. Just around the ruins for a couple of hours, with lots of other tourists around. Then you can go to your cousins." Ted was still trembling.

She paused for a few seconds while she studied his face. "Okay, señor. I come with you."

Ted was elated and smiled for the first time in weeks.

After the train arrived in the village of Machu Picchu, Ted and Corazon boarded a bus for the last leg of the trip, a thirty-minute, winding ride up the mountain to the ruins. They sat together, close to the front. The guide, who was standing at the front of the bus, pointed out the wild orchids that lined the route, but Ted was so smitten with Corazon that he barely noticed them. He could feel his restive heart, but he knew he wasn't ill; it was because he was sitting so close to Corazon. *Does she feel the same way about me? Does she? God, I hope she does. And I pray that she's not already married.*

People were in a great hurry to get off the bus when it arrived at the top, and the guide offered to accompany Ted and Corazon to the site.

They walked for a few minutes, and then Ted stopped short and gave a little gasp. The stunning site was now in full view, surrounded by the awe-inspiring Andes Mountains. The Urubamba River was far below, a tiny silver streak. *This is as close to God as you can get while you're alive. What church can compare to this?*

The guide led Ted and Corazon to the Sun Temple. "The best fitting stones, the best construction was used for the temple," the guide said.

"You speak very good English," Ted exclaimed.

"Thank you, señor. I take evening classes in Cusco." The guide was beaming.

Ted smiled at Corazon. "Where did you learn English?"

"I also take classes and want to learn more. I love English," she said in a firm tone.

Excellent. She loves English. Ted was thrilled.

The guide pointed at a collection of stones close to the temple. "If you look closely, you will see that the stones form the shape of a condor. The condor is a symbol of the higher world, the world above the ground."

"I see it! Yes, I see it." Ted was so excited he wanted to grab Corazon's hand and soar like a condor with her toward the imposing cloud-smothered mountains.

They walked a little further and stopped. "This is the king's palace. See how well the stones fit? Almost as well as at the temple."

Corazon ran toward the palace, stopped at the entrance, and turned to smile at Ted and the guide.

Ted was breathless. He could imagine her dressed in the royal robes of an Inca princess. "May I take your picture?" He quickly got his camera out of his backpack.

"Sure," she said.

Ted took several pictures of Corazon before the guide led them over a rocky path to another group of stone structures.

"Nobles lived in these houses," the guide said with a sweeping gesture.

A little pebble suddenly rolled off a hill overgrown with bushes. Corazon looked up instantly and whispered, "Look! It's a chinchilla."

"It is? Where?" Ted and the guide said together as they strained to see it.

"Close to top, under the biggest bush," Corazon said quietly.

A little brown animal that looked like a cross between a sea otter and a marmot showed itself. It sniffed the air and slowly moved its head from side to side as it cautiously checked them out.

"He is so cute. I want take him home," Corazon said with a broad grin. "My puppies would love him too. I love animals. They love you back. Anything you do for them, they love you."

"Corazon—what a perfect name for you," Ted said slowly and thoughtfully. "You have so much heart, and you're full of love." He trembled as much as he had on the train when he met her.

Corazon noticed the trembling, looked straight into his eyes, and lightly touched his arm.

She cares about me. Maybe the condor heard my wish. Ted loved Corazon's dark eyes.

The guide led them to the terraced areas that had been used for agriculture and then politely told them he had other tourists to take care of. Ted thanked him and gave him a good tip.

When Ted and Corazon arrived back at the site entrance, Ted extended his arm and gave Corazon a sincere look, hoping and praying she would lean on his arm.

She smiled at him, and his prayer was answered. He tingled all over when she took his arm. They boarded one of the buses that was waiting to take tourists back to the village, sat next to each other, and enjoyed the ride back down. The driver was obviously very experienced and careful.

Ted jumped off the bus and held out his hand for Corazon.

"Do you have time for a quick dinner with me before you visit your cousins? Please say yes," Ted pleaded.

"*Si*, I do. I know a good *restaurante* with good tortilla soup," Corazon said cheerfully.

She led him to a café that was quite close to a huge statue of an Inca king in the main square.

I love that. She knows where she's going, and she knows what she wants.

They had a light meal, and then Ted found the courage to give Corazon his hotel address and phone number in Cusco.

"I will be in Cusco for another week. Please call me when you get back. Please." Ted spoke imploringly and touched her arm with infinite tenderness.

Corazon agreed immediately, and Ted was ecstatic.

They walked together to the train station, enjoying the colorful arts and crafts stalls along the way. She stayed with him until he boarded the train and promised to contact him in Cusco.

Ted saw Corazon's beautiful, noble young face in the mountainous landscape all the way back. Even the evening darkness couldn't obscure it.

He didn't sleep much that night, even though he had a comfortable bed in the best hotel close to the cathedral. He rushed down to the lobby in the morning to calm his nerves over breakfast.

He didn't stray too far from the hotel after breakfast and made sure all the clerks knew he was waiting for a young lady to contact him.

Corazon walked through the hotel doors just after Ted finished his lunch in the restaurant close to the lobby. He jumped up from his table and rushed to meet her, nearly knocking a chair over along the way.

"You came, you came." Ted held her arms gently.

She grinned at him and gave him a playful pat on the arm. "You are funny, señor."

Ted led her to a comfortable sofa in a quieter, private part of the lobby.

"Please call me Ted. Please."

"Okay, Ted." She gave a disarming little giggle.

Ted took a very deep breath. He looked into Corazon's eyes and breathed deeply again. "Do you believe in love at first sight? You know, *amor primero vista* or something like that?"

Corazon nodded vigorously.

"Well, it's happened to me." Ted put his warm hand over Corazon's.

"You fall in love with a lady here in Cusco and you want, how you say, advice?" Corazon spoke slowly and deliberately. She was realistic and practical and sounded as if she was willing to help.

Ted took another deep breath before he spoke. "No, I fell in love with a lovely young lady on the train on the way to Machu Picchu. It's you, Corazon. I'm in love with you," he whispered.

Corazon gave a little gasp. "I knew you like me but love? *Amor*? Really?" She looked astounded and thrilled at the same time.

Ted scrutinized her face and saw the thrill in her expression. It gave him the courage to continue. "Corazon, I'm a wealthy man, but I'm very lonely. I'm divorced and don't have a girlfriend waiting for me back home. I must tell you a few things about my life." His voice was low and soft.

"Please tell me." Corazon looked very sincere and concerned.

"I did not come from a happy family." He paused to gaze at her. "I'll bet you do. I'll bet you come from a big, happy family."

"Yes, I do. Big, happy family. We are poor farmers, but we love each other so much. I love my mama and papa and all my brothers and sisters. I do anything for them, they do anything for me. *Mucho amor* in my life." She smiled radiantly.

"You have an amor? A boyfriend?" Ted frowned.

"Non, no boyfriend. Many want me, but I no want them." She laughed.

Ted was so relieved he managed to laugh along with her.

Then he got serious again. "My father was a cold, dangerous man." He sighed long and hard. "When I was eighteen, he pointed a shotgun at me and told me to get out of the house and make my own way in the world. He said that would make a real man out of me. You know, a tough *hombre*."

Corazon drew a sharp breath, and her hand shot up to her mouth. "He do that to you? *Madre de Dios*!"

"Yes, and that was the last time I saw him. My mother died a few years later."

Corazon's eyes grew wider and wider.

"I worked very hard and became highly successful on the outside, but inside I have heart trouble in every way. I have heart palpitations and am very lonely." He took Corazon's other hand. "But … but I know that you are what I have been looking for ever since my father kicked me out. I need you. God, I need you. And I hope you need me just as much."

Corazon shifted closer to him and put her head on his shoulder.

Ted quickly glanced around the room to make sure they were still alone. "You may think I'm crazy, *loco*, but you would bring brilliant light and joy into my life if you would marry me. And I would try very hard to be a good husband. You deserve the best in life."

Corazon moved even closer to him. "How long you stay here? Can you meet my family? Then I decide."

Ted was so excited he jumped in before she finished her last word. "I'll stay as long as it takes! And I want to meet your family, of course."

Corazon introduced Ted to her big, happy family the next day. They treated him very well, as if he were a long-lost cousin. Since they were astute judges of character, Corazon agreed to marry him.

Ted took Corazon back to his lovely home overlooking the beach and shimmering ocean in St. Petersburg. She adjusted to her new life and surroundings immediately, and Ted allowed her to transform the house from nice to stunning by getting rid of ordinary furniture and replacing it with Spanish antiques that could have graced a magnificent hacienda. He gave her expensive jewelry and a good allowance for her clothes and encouraged her to have lots of pets.

She showed her gratitude by cooking gourmet meals and being the perfect housekeeper.

Ted tried hard to be a good husband, but his traumatic past would occasionally overwhelm him and turn him into an ogre. Corazon smothered him with love, and when that wasn't enough to lift him out of his self-induced despair, she left him alone and visited her wonderful family in Cusco.

He would be fine alone for a few days, and then he would call her and beg her to come home.

He remained very ambitious for many years and amassed even more wealth until he was felled by open-heart surgery. No matter how much he grumbled and griped about his condition, Corazon reminded him of how lucky he really was and nursed him as well as any professional nurse.

Ted became very depressed and terribly moody after he recovered from the surgery. He withdrew from social life altogether and lashed out at Corazon as well. She eventually had a mild nervous breakdown, and her doctor gave Ted hell over the phone. He realized that Corazon was too precious a woman to be abused like that and told Ted to smarten up if he wanted to keep her in his life.

After Corazon recovered from her breakdown, Ted vowed to try and be a better person.

When he brought her back from the hospital, he placed her in a throne-like carved chair and got down on his knees in front of her. "Please forgive me, Corazon. I'm so grateful to you for softening my heart. Now I know for sure that money alone isn't enough to cure a damaged heart." He sobbed brokenly, like a little boy who had nearly lost his mother.

"Ted, you always were loco." She stroked his hair gently while the tears streamed down her light brown cheeks. "But I love you anyway, you crazy man."

"You do? You still do?" He put his arms around her knees.

"Si," she whispered. "I wish we could be as happy as we were when we got married."

"I love you just as much as when we met on that train. By God, I do! And I promise to improve from now on and control my nasty moods."

"You better," she said softly.

"I don't know what I'd do without you. I can't live without you."

They held each other for a long time without saying a word.

Chapter 25

Valentine's Day Every Day

Nancy couldn't stand her life in Texas anymore. Her uber-rich husband had recently left her for a younger woman, and her three kids were apathetic toward her. A few friends remained true, but most of them became insufferably condescending and snobby. She was fifty-five and needed a radically new life.

She knew that there had been a horrendous civil war in El Salvador and that over seventy-five thousand innocent people had been killed between 1980 and 1992. In spite of that, quite a few Americans had moved there after the war because of the low cost of living, warm climate, and natural beauty, so she transferred her sizeable divorce settlement to a bank in San Salvador and moved to a comfortable house on the beach close to the city. Before long, she had established a large network of American and Canadian friends who had houses in the city and on the beach. She loved the tropical climate so much that her health improved tremendously, and she spent many hours walking on the beaches and befriending the locals.

The locals in the area came to love her because she opened a nutritious soup kitchen at her home after a horrifically destructive hurricane washed away many nearby roads and bridges; everyone knew that *Señora* Nancy's house was always open and that she wouldn't let anyone starve. She didn't have to worry about crime because the word quickly spread through the grapevine that she was fabulously generous and kind.

A friend from the American Embassy invited her to a Mayan temple ceremony one afternoon. Nancy wore a long white beach dress and pinned a couple of luscious red flowers in her long brown hair. *Something magical is going to happen at the temple. I better look prepared for it.*

As she and her friend walked over the grass toward the pyramidal temple in the outskirts of the city, they heard someone playing a slow, ancient melody on a flute. There were a few dozen people there already, many of them with obvious Mayan heritage. Their large, almond-shaped eyes and aquiline noses reminded Nancy of carvings she had seen in local museums. Nancy and her friend strolled through the crowd, anxious to get a good look at the flute player.

"There he is," Nancy's friend whispered. "Look at the gorgeous Mayan costume. He looks like a temple priest. And the feather hanging from his ear. And he's young and handsome too. Aren't you glad we came?"

"Sure am," Nancy said.

The flute player finished his melody soon after the women arrived in front of him.

He smiled, gave a gentle bow, and said, "I am Chico. And you?"

Nancy and her friend introduced themselves.

Chico, who was muscular and agile, with long black hair pulled back in a ponytail, led them to a bench at the periphery of the ceremonial area. "I am Mayan. Many, many years ago." He threw his hand back to indicate that he was Mayan for many generations.

Nancy and her friend nodded with enthusiasm.

"During Civil War, I … I was … forced … to kill." He pretended to be using a machine gun. "I was forced to kill good … good people. If I no do it …" He pretended to slit his own throat. "If I no do it, the generales they tell me they kill my family."

"Oh, my God …" Nancy and her friend said at once.

"Now, to forget war, I am guide here at temple. I teach about Mayan life." He picked up a thick, round, jade-turquoise stone disc. "This is Mayan calendar," he said with great reverence, as if it were his most prized possession.

"Oh, and the Mayans said the world will end in 2012?" Nancy asked, raising her eyebrows.

"No." Chico shook his head. "New cycle. Not end, just new cycle." He grinned.

Nancy and her friend were impressed with the intricately carved disc full of mysterious symbols. They traced some of the symbols with their fingers.

"You like? I teach you about ancient Mayan wisdom one day."

A group of men and women in Mayan costumes approached them. "You … you are Nancy!" One of the ladies smiled at her. "We know about you. You feed people after the hurricane. You don't look like us, but you have a Mayan heart."

Nancy drew a sharp breath of appreciation. "Thank you, thank you! That's the best compliment I could possibly get." She was so elated that she was breathless.

"I know too." Chico gave her an admiring look and spoke with a warm, firm tone.

If only my ex could see me now. Here I am, the center of attention in a beautiful spiritual ceremony and rising to a higher level of consciousness.

Three older men dressed in long white robes knelt and touched the earth close to the temple.

"Earth is wisdom," Chico murmured as he watched them with affectionate eyes.

"And even though we live in modern society, we Mayans admire these wise men and talk to them frequently to get guidance," one of the friendly ladies said. "I am an accountant, but I admire my wise man. He is a farmer, but he is far wiser than I am."

Everyone felt like a cherished child of the universe by the time the ceremony finished.

Nancy's American friend noticed that Chico and Nancy were kindred spirits; she wanted to give them some privacy, so she left with some other friends. Nancy drove Chico back to her place, and the two sat under a tall palm tree on the beach and talked all night over the ocean waves that gently slapped the sand.

By morning, they were best friends, and the misty pink dawn seemed to bless them.

They began working as a team to buy school supplies for underfunded schools. They looked for teachers who were willing to spend extra time with the kids and give them a chance to succeed. They organized social events for young people, and they worked with the San Salvador elite to help orphans. A few El Salvadoreans were incredibly wealthy, but too many were so heartbreakingly poor that they could not afford to raise their children and were forced to abandon them at orphanages.

A Valentine's Day lunch party at a huge, hacienda-like cultural center with arched hallways, polished floors, and ornately carved Spanish furniture was planned for a large group of orphans. Round tables were set up to display the handicrafts the children had made, and the city elite were encouraged to buy as many of these wares as possible so the orphanages would get extra funds. The children were taught skills that would eventually help them find jobs. Red, heart-shaped balloons were attached to all the tables in the large room that was reserved for the fundraiser.

There were a few orphaned boys dressed in neat shirts and pants, but most of the orphans were girls in pink dresses. Most were about twelve years old, give or take a year or two. They were so well behaved and had such pleasant dispositions that it was hard to believe they were orphans. They stood patiently by the handicraft tables and waited for people to buy their goods. Several young nuns in simple light beige habits helped to coordinate their activities.

When the time for buying handicrafts was over, everyone sat down for lunch. The whole room was vibrating with excitement and goodwill, so much so that the chief organizer of the fundraiser had to repeatedly ask everyone to calm down and listen. When she could be heard, the organizer announced that a good deal of money was raised for the orphanages. Everyone clapped wildly, and then there was an announcement about three well-known local musicians who were to perform during lunch. Everyone was instantly and totally quiet.

An elegant mature lady singer and two silver-haired men with guitars appeared. They sang slowly, graciously, and with the delicacy of love itself:

Amor, amor, amor, this word so sweet, that I repeat, means
I adore you.
Amor, amor, my love, would you deny this heart that I
Have placed before you.

When they finished singing that famous song, everyone cheered. Many said they had never heard it performed so beautifully and with so much unspeakable tenderness. There were many moist eyes in the audience; everyone knew that this song was meant to touch the hearts of the orphans.

They performed more lovely songs with exquisite, spellbinding musicianship.

Then CDs of fantastically lively Latin dance music were played, and everyone, including the nuns and the orphans, got up to dance around the room. Someone shouted, "We should have Valentine's Day every day!"

Someone else shouted, "We do, we do!"

Nancy, Chico, and everyone else who wanted to help economically disadvantaged children were frequent visitors to Miguel Angel Ramirez's studio in the picturesque village of Panchimalco. Children went to his studio, which was an older elegant house with a lovely multilevel garden, for art lessons. The internationally renowned Miguel and his colleagues tried to help the kids express themselves through art, and Miguel's paintings of children with enormously wide eyes seem to symbolize the new zeitgeist, the renewed collective soul of El Salvador. They expressed a longing to forget the tragic past and look forward to a peaceful new life overflowing with the sweet innocence of childhood. One could say that the rest of the world needs a similar healing experience!

Nancy rarely looked back to her previous life anymore—the time when her self-confidence was lower. People told her she wouldn't survive alone in El Salvador, but she knew they were wrong and that she belonged there; she was helping the locals regain their faith in humanity and thereby blossoming into the woman she was always meant to be.

* * * * *

Nancy had a big party one evening, and everyone was invited. I enjoyed talking to a whole spectrum of types of people, but I was saddened when a group of young local men told me that they felt uneasy around some of the wealthy American and Canadian men.

They said these men had been brainwashed for years with the idea that the cream of society were the lighter-skinned people, the ones in the middle level were mixtures of whites and natives, and the ones at the very bottom were the indigenous descendants of the Mayans. I had seen a museum display in San Salvador to that effect. The colonial elite were those of pure Spanish extraction, and the more native blood one had, the lower the social status. Some of these men had lived and worked in the States for a few years, got used to a more egalitarian society, and had mixed feelings about being forced to return home.

Wayne, who was a loveable big bear of a retired American businessman and who had a cottage on the beach not too far from Nancy's house and an apartment in the city, never made anyone feel uncomfortable. He was perfectly at peace with himself, always cheerful, helpful, and confident, and the locals felt great around him. He glided easily from one group to another at the party and made everyone laugh. When he felt that one of the richer guys was showing off too much, he would wiggle his behind at him and say, "*Bésame culo*." Wayne could get away with things like that.

A buxom, older native lady who had been hired to serve drinks approached Wayne with a big bottle of red wine and asked him if he wanted a refill. He grinned and shook his head, but she poured him a full glass anyway. "Ahh, *muchacha malo*! Bad girl!" He spoke with a booming voice, wagged his finger, and pretended to be annoyed with her.

She gave him a mock scowl, which melted when he blew kisses at her. One could see her shoulders shaking with laughter when she walked over to some other guests with the bottle; she was married and was old enough to be a grandmother.

Wayne beckoned me, walked closer to the beach, and sat down next to some local men.

I followed him and sat down across from him.

"Would you like to come to the street party this Friday night?" Wayne gave me a hopeful look.

"This Friday? And where?" I was puzzled because I wasn't sure what he meant.

"We've organized a street party for the young people in the beach area. It will be just a couple of streets over from here, and a DJ will play music so they can dance. They need some fun, and they always enjoy the parties."

Wayne's cell phone rang. "Excuse me for a second," he said while he checked it. "Oh, that's *El Diablo*. He can wait," he said, chuckling as he ignored the call.

"El Diablo?" I snickered.

"He's an old buddy. He lives in the city, and we go to ballgames together. He lived in Boston for years and worked as a mechanic. Whenever anyone around here needs their car fixed, they go to him, and he gives them a good rate because of me." He shoved the cell phone aside and had a gulp of red wine. "Anyway, please come to the party."

"Of course. That's not something any old tourist would experience," I chirped.

Wayne's cell rang again, and he rolled his eyes, pretending to be irritated. He looked at the number. "This time it's *El Hombre Viejo*—the old man."

The young men overhead him and laughed like kids.

"He can wait too."

"Who's he?" I gave him an inquiring look.

"He lives in Costa Rica and knows everybody in Central America. He knows that I'm still using my American driver's license and that I need to get a local ID pronto before the police haul me in for questioning, so he's pulling strings to get me a temporary ID." Wayne sounded totally unfazed.

"The police could haul you in? Oh boy. I've seen the machine guns they have." I shivered.

Wayne gave a long, hearty belly laugh, and one of the young locals said, "Wayne, he no scared of nothing." The group continued their uproarious laughter.

"Oh yeah. Sometimes they stop me for questioning when I'm driving." He paused to giggle. "I pretend I don't know Spanish, and then I keep on driving."

"That's too much," I said.

"I never show them any papers, and I tell them, '*No habla español, lo siento.*'"

"God, what I'd give to have that kind of courage." I shook my head and smiled.

"That's what happens to you when you have to jump out of planes," Wayne said in a pleasant, matter-of-fact tone. "I was a paratrooper for a few years."

I was slack-jawed. "I couldn't do that if my life depended on it."

"Oh yeah, you could." He sounded really sincere, making me feel capable and special. *That's one of the signs of a real leader.*

Wayne came over to Nancy's house on Friday night and accompanied us to the street party. We strolled over the bumpy dirt roads between the beach houses, admiring the moonlit white, yellow, and orange tropical flowers and listening to the distant dance music. "Sounds like a happy crowd," I said.

There was a small covered stage at one end of the street. The DJ was working under a flashing strobe light, and at least fifty people were there. Some were dancing, others were sipping beer and watching the action from a comfortable distance under the trees, and others were milling around the refreshment stand. We bought admission tickets from a young lady who spoke perfect English.

A couple of policemen nodded and smiled at Wayne as he led me and Nancy to the dance area. "I know those two," Wayne said. "They're wondering how I managed to have a beautiful lady on each arm."

Nancy recognized another neighbor and went to dance with

him. Wayne and I danced together and enjoyed being surrounded by youthful energy.

I chuckled. "Look at that guy with the tight white jeans. His legs are as thin as cigarettes, and can he move." The teenage boy, who was about fourteen or fifteen, was gyrating like Elvis in front of his male partner.

Wayne gave me a slight knowing smile as he held my hand. "The other kids call him 'Sissy Boy.' He's having a good time now, but he's in real danger most of the time."

"Uh-oh. Why?"

Wayne turned me around, and when I faced him again, he said, "It's a real macho culture here. The guys don't understand gays. He's been badly beaten on the way to school. I just hope they don't gang up on him and beat the life out of him the next time."

My jaw dropped, and I gasped. "The poor guy."

Wayne nodded. "He knows I'll protect him when I'm around. He came over to my place one day after he'd been beaten. I patched him up, and we had a really good talk. And I'm friends with all the local police, and we work together."

"I'm glad somebody's looking out for him." *Wayne is macho enough to jump out of planes, but he's a real sweetheart. He's just what this place needs—someone humorous, kind, protective, and generous.*

"May I kiss you?" Wayne asked, raising his eyebrows.

I smiled and glanced at the other dancers. "Wait until we leave," I whispered.

"Okay."

Nancy, Wayne, and I left the party at a little after midnight. We could still hear the music on the way back, and after Nancy unlocked her front door and went inside, Wayne gave me a light and tender kiss.

"I think I love you," he whispered.

I think I love you too.

Chapter 26

Love Has the Last Word

While I was facilitating a grief support group for people who were grieving some sort of loss (some had lost spouses, some parents, and some children), I tried to ease their pain by urging them to stand in front of a mirror and say, "I love you." I wanted them to concentrate on their own healing and to treat themselves as holy vessels. They all promised to try that after they got home later in the afternoon.

When we met again a week later, they all told me that they could not say, "I love you." Self-criticism got in the way, and they could not suppress their automatic negative thoughts. (Dr. Daniel Amen, in his book, *Change Your Brain, Change Your Life*, calls these thoughts ants.[17]) One man said he "got a fright" when he looked at himself, and one lady said she could only see her facial flaws and turned her head away from the mirror in disgust.

Many other people have told me the same thing. They would

---

[17] Dr. Daniel Amen, *Change Your Brain, Change Your Life* (New York: Three Rivers Press, 1998).

not be able to say, "I love you" to their mirror image. In my opinion, the people who love themselves enough to be able to do that seem to be exceptional.

When I was a teenager, I read many Western philosophy books. Even though some of them were depressing because they questioned the meaning of life and had no positive answer, the philosophical mind-set sharpened my intellect and urged me to question everything and not blindly and automatically accept the status quo in any facet of life.

For example, when society insists that the most beautiful and desirable women are movie stars or skeletally thin supermodels, one can demolish that standard by using the Socratic method—one can keep asking, "Why?" Eventually one will see that the impossible standard is just another cruel form of judgment that makes most women feel imperfect. Good character, brains, wisdom, compassion, altruism, and other wonderful qualities don't seem to count nearly as much as physical beauty. Why? Why are women not often loved and accepted for their inner beauty? When girls as young as nine have anorexia because they believe they won't be loved if they're not thin, we know our judgments are far too harsh. Even though there is a recent movement away from models being too young and too thin, women are still instantly judged by their age and appearance.

One could use the same method to demolish impossible standards for men. Why must they be supersmart, rich, powerful, and athletic to be fully valued? Is it because they'll pass on their superior genes to their children? Are these genes really superior? What does superior really mean? Supremely brilliant minds developed nuclear weapons, but the only creatures that would survive a global nuclear holocaust would be the cockroaches. Are the superrich really superior in a world of overpopulation and shrinking resources? No matter how rich you are, all you've done is build a bigger sandcastle on the beach of time. You may enjoy it for a while until the waves roll in, smash it, and redistribute the sand. A homeless person could later walk on the same beach and see no trace of your fabulous castle. I feel sorry for the young men I saw on a television program about China; many were heartbroken because they were dumped by their fiancées for not being rich.

We judge each other constantly, spending far too much time playing this cruel game. In some cases, it resembles a blood sport. Are we that bored with our lives? Shouldn't we all be concentrating on making life nicer for everyone else? No wonder the scientists' doomsday clock is always so close to midnight.

I received a copy of Bertrand Russell's *A History of Western Philosophy*[18] for my seventeenth birthday and loved it. I also read books about existentialism, nihilism, and Spinoza. I'm a big-picture or "wholistic" learner, and I like to grasp the macro aspects of anything before I spend time trying to understand the micro or detailed aspects. I favor the "everything in a nutshell" approach. I tried to fathom why there had been a terrible world war just a few years before I was born; why so many millions of innocent people were killed; why there were so many condescending and judgmental people in my upmarket entrepreneurial, professorial, and academic neighborhood; and why there was so much discontent in the midst of obvious and conspicuous wealth and achievement.

Brain scientists have recently shown that the teenage brain is still changing so much that it is unstable.[19] As a teenager, I was not ready to read books about metaphysical nihilism, which question the reality of existence itself. I felt as if I was engulfed by a totally black hole.

Until a little angel changed my life.

---

[18] Bertrand Russell, *A History of Western Philosophy* (New York: Simon and Schuster, 1972).
[19] "The New Science of the Teenage Brain," *National Geographic*, October 2011.

When I was a first-year university science student, I went to the birthday party of a little girl who was twelve years younger than I was. There were many other girls there, along with their mothers, and we were out in the backyard. One of the mothers asked the birthday girl to do something she didn't want to do, and she stomped her foot down with lively determination and cried, "No!" She stomped again. "No!" I was standing right beside her and felt the tremendous energy of her foot stomp. Then she grinned at me and grabbed my hand, saying, "I love you. You're my favorite babysitter, and I wish you were my second mom." In that magical moment, the life force started rushing back into my body. *My God, I really am happy to be alive, and there really is meaning and purpose in the world.* The girl's love was so powerful that it overwhelmed me and energized me, recharging the dead battery of my soul and shining into the black hole of nihilism.

Whether we understand the universe or not, we can improve our lives and find joy by loving and accepting each other. Jesus and other spiritual leaders were right about the ability of love and light to engulf the black hole of despair. People who have faith in a loving source energy have an easier time loving and accepting themselves and others. They know that judging themselves and others too harshly is not necessary for the survival of the species and only leads to hell on earth. Love and light exist, but they have to struggle to shine through the thick jungle of human life.

Logic and research in education and psychology also tell us that society functions better when people are loved and valued. When I was studying education at Louisiana State University in Shreveport, one of my professors told my class that cooperative learning is often better than learning alone or even in pairs. To prove his point, he divided us into some groups of four, some pairs, and some singles and gave us some math problems to solve. The groups found the solutions faster every time. When people feel loved, accepted, and valued, they perform at their best. What a world this would be if we would love and accept each other and work together toward positive common goals!

Imagine a sports team comprised of seven billion members, all having different jobs but all working toward the same goal. It's hard enough just trying to stay alive on this planet; we need all the positive, concerted energy we can muster to survive as a species. Why should we waste valuable energy judging, excluding, and fighting members of the same team? Constructive criticism should be the norm; we don't need destructive criticism. In spite of the fact that we are biologically programmed to be territorial and competitive, it's time to build a kinder, gentler, more evolved version of society. Life on earth depends on it.

Before I was allowed to start my first teaching job, I was required to see a film called *The Self-Fulfilling Prophecy*. When people are treated with genuine respect and are expected to shine, they often rise to the occasion and behave in a way that deserves that respect. As new teachers, we were told to expect nothing but the best from our students and to treat them with respect. Criticizing the child himself or herself was forbidden, but we could offer constructive criticism to alter undesirable *behavior*.

Adults are just like kids; they rise to the occasion when they feel appreciated and valued.

So many situations in life are win/lose because the world is so greedy and competitive. Some are winners, but many are losers. However, when people love and accept themselves and others and don't waste valuable energy judging each other, the situation becomes win/win. The world would be transformed overnight if we all suddenly decided to stand in front of a mirror and say, "I love you" and really mean it. You must love yourself before you can truly love others.

All the major religions emphasize the power of God's love for us. Huston Smith, in his classic book, *The World's Religions*,[20] tells us that Jews believe we are a blend of dust and divinity and that people are God's beloved children. Islam tells us that in the sight of the Lord all people are equal. Hindus think that the point of life is to transcend the smallness of the finite self and that never during its pilgrimage is the human spirit completely adrift and alone. The transpersonal God is the sole ground of human existence and awareness. Christians believe that God has an overwhelming love of humanity, and Jesus tried to convey God's absolute love for every single human being. Buddha was born for the good of many, out of compassion for the world, and the Dalai Lama's function is to incarnate on earth the celestial principle of compassion and mercy.

In 2011, I read a pithy BBC Internet news article[21] that says it all. According to the article, social scientists conducted a worldwide study and found that *lack of self-esteem is at the root of most mental health problems, and there are millions and millions of people with mental health problems, especially anxiety and depression.* Hordes of people are on antidepressants and tranquilizers, and I personally know some people who have tried to commit suicide because they have very low self-esteem and feel that they are not worthy of love.

According to the researchers quoted by the BBC, there are a few things you should do to stay mentally healthy: Take the time to relax and enjoy yourself, be with friends and have fun, do physical activities like sports, and organize your time to feel "on top" of tasks. Every day, think about what you like about yourself. Have a thoughtful, compassionate attitude to yourself, like you would with a friend, and laugh. Find the funny things in life, because humor is good for physical and mental health.

The BBC also discussed a recent worldwide study on happiness

---

20 Huston Smith, *The World's Religions* (New York: HarperCollins, 1986).
21 James Tighe, "Low Self-Esteem," BBC Online, www.bbc.co.uk/health/emotional_health/mental_health/emotion_esteem.shtml, BBC Online.

that showed people are happiest when having a face-to-face conversation with a friendly person, having a romance, or exercising. Our mental health depends very much on positive interactions with others.

Frank Minirth, MD, and Paul Meier, MD, wrote a marvelous bestseller titled *Happiness Is a Choice*.[22] The last chapter informs us how to find lifelong happiness, and one of the most important things you can do is to *change the way you talk to yourself.* If you constantly criticize yourself, you'll hold grudges against yourself and get depressed. Quit condemning yourself. Instead, look at the positive things in your life. Look at your accomplishments instead of dwelling on past failures. Would you ever criticize another person as much as you subconsciously criticize yourself? You may think you need all that harsh talk, but you don't—so get off your back!

Depression raises cortisol levels, and that can suppress lymphocytes (certain white blood cells), which produce antibodies. With fewer antibodies, one becomes more susceptible to nearly all physical illnesses. Depression is pent-up anger, and the authors of *Happiness Is a Choice* think that *pent-up anger is the leading cause of death.*

Matthew McKay, PhD, and Patrick Fanning wrote a classic book on self-esteem titled *Self-Esteem*.[23] They tell us that self-esteem is an attitude of acceptance and not being judgmental toward self and others. They recommend doing a self-concept inventory divided into the following categories: your physical appearance, how you relate to others, your personality, how others see you, your performance on the job, your performance of daily tasks of life, your mental functioning, and your sexuality. They suggest you write down all the

---

[22] Frank Minirth and Paul Meier, *Happiness Is a Choice* (Grand Rapids, MI: Baker Books, 2007).
[23] Matthew McKay and Patrick Fanning, *Self-Esteem* (Oakland, CA: New Harbinger Publications, 2000).

positive and negative things you can think of under each heading. However, you are not to use harshly critical language to emphasize what you think are negative qualities. *Be kind to yourself, even when describing your undesirable characteristics.*

When you are finished, combine your strengths and weaknesses into a self-description that is accurate, fair, and supportive. It will acknowledge weaknesses that you might like to change, but it will also include the personal assets that are an integral part of your identity. They also suggest using these affirmations: *I love myself. I am confident. I am successful. I do my best. I am interested in life. I am fine just the way I am.*

Now go and stand in front of a mirror and say, "I love you."